# OVERCOMING CANCER

### Exposing Toxic Enemies of the Spirit, Soul, and Body

# OVERCOMING CANCER

## Exposing Toxic Enemies of the Spirit, Soul, and Body

### Gretchen Ostrom

WINEPRESS WP PUBLISHING

© 2001 by Covenant Ministry. All rights reserved.

Printed in the United States of America.

Packaged by WinePress Publishing, PO Box 428, Enumclaw, WA 98022. The views expressed or implied in this work do not necessarily reflect those of WinePress Publishing. Ultimate design, content, and editorial accuracy of this work are the responsibility of the author.

No part of this publication may be reproduced, stored in a retrieval system or transmitted in any way by any means, electronic, mechanical, photocopy, recording or otherwise, without the prior permission of the copyright holder except as provided by USA copyright law.

Unless otherwise noted, all Scriptures are taken from the Holy Bible, New International Version, Copyright © 1973, 1978, 1984 by the International Bible Society. Used by permission of Zondervan Publishing House. The "NIV" and "New International Version" trademarks are registered in the United States Patent and Trademark Office by International Bible Society.

Verses marked TLB are taken from The Living Bible, Copyright © 1971 owned by assignment by Illinois Regional Bank N.A. (as trustee). Used by permission of Tyndale House Publishers, Inc., Wheaton, Illinois 60189. All rights reserved.

ISBN 1-57921-371-5
Library of Congress Catalog Card Number: 2001 087748

# Acknowledgments

This book is dedicated first and foremost to the One who made it all possible and is the inspiration for the testimony within these pages. This journey began with the promise that I was going to live and that this journey would be a testimony and tribute to the goodness of God and that the Son of God, the Lord Jesus Christ would be glorified in it. I am eternally indebted to the mercy and grace of God for allowing me to become part of the household of faith through the atoning sacrifice of His son, the Lord Jesus Christ.

My beloved sons, Matthew and Joseph have been a source of motivation and encouragement when facing what seemed like hopeless obstacles. Matthew, my first-born, was always willing to help me research any medical issue and find information on Medline. Thankfully he could translate the medical "tech talk" into language I could understand. You will be a wonderful physician Matt and I know our experience has only served to help you appreciate the complex issues every physician needs to understand including the spiritual and emotional components to healing. You will be a skilled, wise and compassionate physician one day. Thank you for the countless hours of patient listening and unwavering strength you gave me.

My dear Joseph your tender-hearted kindness and gentleness was always like the balm of Gilead pouring over my soul—great medicine—better than chicken soup. Thank you for all the generous compassion you showered upon me all these years as we patiently waited for the promised blessing. You were always consistent

# Overcoming Cancer

and steadfastly hopeful, encouraging me when I was down. Your sweet presence always brings refreshment to my heart.

This book is to help you better understand the loving, intimate relationship available to you with your heavenly Father. May you come to treasure the word of God as his loving instruction and guidance for you in all your ways. Moses wrote in Deuteronomy 6:5–7 "Love the Lord your God with all your heart and with all your soul and with all your strength. These commandments that I give you today are to be upon your hearts. Impress them on your children. Talk about them when you sit at home and when you walk along the road, when you lie down and when you get up." This will be your greatest accomplishment when you have successfully transmitted this heritage to future generations.

My heartfelt thanks and appreciation are extended to my editor Margaret Smith, author of *Journal Keeper*, as she encouraged me in the writing process.

> *The word of God is living and active. Sharper than any double-edged sword, it penetrates even to dividing soul and spirit, joints and marrow; it judges the thoughts and attitudes of the heart. Nothing in all creation is hidden from God's sight. Everything is uncovered and laid bare before the eyes of him to whom we must give account.*
> —Hebrews 4:12–13

In Loving Memory of

**Dr. Glenn Warner**
July 11, 1919–November 11, 2000

He was the hands of the Great Physician here on earth. Although scorned, ridiculed and condemned by his colleagues he persevered and continued to love and inspire his patients. Dr. Glenn Warner provided faith when I did not have it, courage to go on and medical wisdom to enable me to overcome a cancer battle.

"Well done" Dr. Warner, you have been a good and faithful servant and I know you have received your reward. I am blessed and enriched to have known you.

# Contents

Introduction .................................................................. x

Lessons from the Furnace ............................................. 16
    A Doctor's Report, or the Report of the Lord? ................... 19

Inquire of the Lord ....................................................... 25
    Identify the Enemy and Learn the Tactics ....................... 30

The Detoxification Process ........................................... 36

Nutritional Supplementation ......................................... 40
    Table of Supplements and Nutritional Support ................ 42

Spiritual Healing .......................................................... 48

Working Out My Salvation . . . One Day at a Time .......... 54
    Personal reflection: ...................................................... 67

Emotional Healing ....................................................... 70
    My Father's Heart ........................................................ 70
    The Art of Hope .......................................................... 74

# Contents

Continue to Persevere ..................................................... 76
    Power of Praise ............................................................ 79

Job's Friends
    Come to Visit ............................................................ 83

Physical Healing ............................................................... 90
    How Could Things Get Worse? ........................................ 90

Peace at Last ..................................................................... 96

Appendix ........................................................................ 103
    Healing Prayer According to God's Word ...................... 103

Cancer is Limited ......................................................... 116

Detoxification Techniques: Some Friendly Advice .......... 117
    The Famous and Therapeutic Coffee Enema .................. 117
    Sauna Regimen ........................................................... 118
    Hydrotherapy at Home (from Healing Naturally) ........... 119

Recommended Reading and References ....................... 122

# Introduction

My original intention for writing about my journey of healing was to leave a testimony, as a memorial of God's faithfulness, for my sons and their families. I hope it will serve as a legacy for them to cherish, so they will know their God, his goodness, kindness and great mercy. In 2 Samuel 7:12, after the Israelites defeat the Philistines, Samuel erects a monument to the Lord and calls it Ebenezer, saying, "Thus far the Lord has helped us." Just as the Israelites erected a monument to the Lord to honor him, this testimony is my Ebenezer, my acknowledgment of God's goodness. Notice that the words were, "Thus far the Lord has helped us," and so it is that the Lord is faithful and will continue to help his children in the days to come. May my sons, grandchildren, and future generations come to know his faithfulness and loving kindness to them as they journey through this life.

Here is another reason I wrote this book. Over the years, I have met many people struggling with illness, chronic disease and life threatening situations. A number of these people have asked me how I have managed during this season of life, where I have battled cancer for over eight years. In response to these requests, I have decided to document the lessons God has taught me through this process, to provide encouragement and hope for others. It is heartbreaking to see so many people who do not realize the healthcare options available.

We live in a world so full of toxins that in the days ahead, it will require a concerted effort to maintain excellent health. I have learned how to battle for God's promised blessings of health and well-being, and I do believe that it is a battle. In order to be healthy,

## Introduction

we must be equipped for the future. I hope that I can provide you with some keys to healthy living.

Since the beginnings of my struggle with cancer, I have become more keenly aware how essential the word of God is, how valuable his precepts and commandments. God does not show favoritism. His promises are for all who would call upon his name. He has not left us alone and without hope, like helpless victims. What he promised in his word is available to all who believe.

I would not want to imply that I know all the dynamics of healing for each reader, because each of us is an individual, with a different history and different life experiences. God deals with each of us personally, not only spiritually but also physically and in our soul (mind, will and emotions). He will reveal the path of healing for each of us as we seek his counsel. When we are sick, it only makes sense to seek out the Great Physician and trust our lives completely to him. God alone knows the roots of our diseases, the innermost parts of our being and the intricacies of our lives since our conception. Who, apart from our Creator, can best determine a course of treatment and devise a strategy for us to regain our balance and well-being?

Because we live in a sinful, broken world, we are subject to the consequences of this life. We live with our own shortcomings and those of others. But God restores, heals and makes us prosper in his kingdom. Although we suffer here, we can still know the power of the Resurrection and the miracle of his loving intervention in our lives.

It is faith that pleases God. Throughout my life with God, my prayer has always been that I would be pleasing to him. Little did I know what refining fire I would have to go through in order to grow in my faith. I know according to what is written in the Bible that there is a purpose in suffering and in trials. As Paul says in Romans 5:3–5,

> *So we also rejoice in our sufferings, because we know that suffering produces perseverance; perseverance, character; and character, hope. And hope does not disappoint us, because God*

*has poured out his love into our hearts by the Holy Spirit, whom he has given us.*

And as the Bible tells us in James 1:2–4,

*Consider it pure joy, my brothers, whenever you face trials of many kinds, because you know that the testing of your faith develops perseverance, perseverance must finish its work so that you may be mature and complete, not lacking anything. If any of you lacks wisdom, he should ask God, who gives generously to all without finding fault, and it will be given to him . . . . Blessed is the man who perseveres under trial, because when he has stood the test, he will receive the crown of life that God has promised to those who love him.*

See all the benefits of these trials: joy, which becomes a choice, not based on circumstances; perseverance; character; hope; wisdom; faith; humility; love; and the reward from the Lord, the crown of life. That is good news for those who are suffering and enduring trials. We are always in the process of transformation in our innermost being, going from faith to faith by God's grace.

I have come to understand that there are at least two concepts that determine victory and fruitfulness in the life of a Christian. The first concept is that the Lord wants us free from bondage, past hurts, lies, misconceptions, false beliefs and childish behaviors. Secondly, he wants us to reach maturity, being conformed to the likeness of Jesus. God wants to perfect the church in holiness, purity and unity.

It is through this process of testing, trials and suffering that we choose to grow and mature. Please note that I carefully chose the word *choose*. We may opt out, of course, and miss all that the Lord has destined for us. Tried integrity is a state of mind that has stood the test. One who remains under trials in a God-honoring way, rather than escaping them in order to be relieved of the pressure, is able to learn the lessons those trials are sent to teach. This season of trial and testing for me has led me to a deeper examination of the depths of sin in my heart, as well as a departure from my

# Introduction

self-sufficiency and self-righteousness. It has been a time of earnest wrestling with God in prayer. It has been his sustaining grace that has given me strength and renewed hope.

As Paul worshipped and grasped a momentary glimpse of God's purposes, he is overcome by the illumination of God's character and says, "Oh, the depth of the riches of the wisdom and knowledge of God. How unsearchable his judgments, and his paths beyond tracing out!"

I can echo those thoughts with praise, because of the ways God has orchestrated my life. He has caused circumstances, whether good or evil, to be transformed for his purpose and, ultimately, for his glory. The word *transform* means to change completely or essentially in composition and structure. Now, that is a major construction project to undertake. Fortunately, God has left us examples of those who have gone before and left their testimonies as examples to encourage us, as we see God working in their lives.

For example, in the book of Genesis, we see that Joseph's life was replete with what could have been devastating circumstances and the ruin of a young man. His own brothers cast him into a pit to die. He was rescued, only to face slavery, imprisonment, betrayal and false accusations. Joseph could have justified an attitude of bitterness and anger toward God. But he continued, by faith, to trust in the Almighty. After years of hardship, Joseph was rewarded for his faith, reaching a place of international influence, leadership and prosperity. Joseph's attitude is reflected in his words to his brothers: "As for you, you meant evil against me, but God meant it for good in order to bring about this present result, to preserve many people alive." By now Joseph was settled in his heart that God was sovereign. All Joseph's experiences only served a greater purpose. God is a good God, always seeking to redeem people from destruction and moving miraculously in the lives of his servants.

Who would have thought that the dysfunction of an alcoholic home could be used for God's good purpose for others? How could the diagnosis of a terminal illness, with no known medical cure and a maximum life expectancy of three years, possibly bring God glory? At first, my only perspective of these situations was that

# Overcoming Cancer

they were a source of much sorrow and suffering. How could a commitment to Christ cause such alienation between family members and be such a source of anguish and agony? Paradoxically, they have served to bring me to a more intimate relationship with my Lord. All of these trials have indeed been purposeful and not without profit. It is very difficult, in the midst of the pain and distress, to see a purpose at the time.

But now that I have come through the healing process associated with these situations, I can look back and see the wisdom and lessons I have learned. Now I can see how God has taken these seemingly destructive influences and caused them to work for my good. I hope the examples of God's goodness to me will be an encouragement to others, because what he has done for me he is always willing to do for all his children. God is a good, loving Father who desires our healing, restoration and prosperity.

Many people have helped me in my journey of healing and deliverance by praying, and by encouraging and loving me. Now, in turn, I want to instill a sense of hope to you who may be facing insurmountable circumstances that seem desperate. Sometimes God brings us to the place where there is no human deliverance or means of escape, in order to show himself strong and mighty on our behalf. Nothing is impossible with God.

Today as I say that, it is not simply a mental assent but a deep-down, heartfelt belief. When Job reached the end of his trials and tragedies, he could say that he no longer had heard about God's mighty deeds but he had seen and known them for himself. Job went from a faith that not only *believed* that God can do what he has promised. Now Job *knew* God would do so. I, too, feel privileged to know my God in a personal and intimate way, and for me this intimacy could only have come from a place of complete desperation and need.

I had always been a resourceful, self-sufficient person, but God wanted me to know how sufficient he is. He allowed me to come to the end of my resources and my abilities, so that in my limitations I began to know him as the one in whom there is absolutely no limitation. It is by him alone that I have learned to overcome. The blessings of well-being are promised for all of us, but it has become necessary to contend for those promised blessings. The healing and deliverance has been a process that has served to build me in ways I would never have realized, had my healing been an instantaneous miracle. Learning to contend and persevere, growing in faith and knowing my God has made the journey more than worth the effort. Stay in the battle, and never lose hope.

# Lessons from the Furnace

More than eight years ago, I was diagnosed with multiple myeloma, a malignant form of bone marrow cancer. The Holy Spirit spoke very clearly to me then, saying that I would be learning some important lessons from this. First he said I would need to hear the voice of the Lord, because in the days ahead my life might depend upon it. That was a sobering message. I desperately want to be like a lamb who hears the voice of her Good Shepherd, knowing how I am prone to wander or, more often than I like to admit, am simply aloof. In John 10:1–10 Jesus says:

> I tell you the truth, the man who does not enter the sheep pen by the gate, but climbs in by some other way, is a thief and a robber. The man who enters by the gate is the shepherd of his sheep. The watchman opens the gate for him and the sheep listen to his voice. He calls his own sheep by name and leads them out. When he has brought out all his own, he goes on ahead of them and his sheep follow him because they know his voice. But they will never follow a stranger; in fact, they will run away from him because they do not recognize a stranger's voice.

Many voices in our society today clamor for attention. There is only one voice I need to listen to. Life will go well for me as I trust more in following my Shepherd: God, the lover of my soul.

In addition to hearing God's voice, the Holy Spirit told me he was going to teach me more about spiritual warfare. He would teach me how to be strong and healthy in my physical body, and I would become strong and steadfast in character. All these things were a necessary part of his plan for me in anticipation for the days to come. Now, this was a provocative message. My first reaction was, "How can I get out of this? It feels like too heavy a burden to bear!"

Where do you turn, when faced with these circumstances? I tried everything I could conceive of to avoid all this trial, looking for a way of escape! The reality began to sink in. All I could do was to cast myself on the Lord and cry for mercy and help, saying, "Here I am Lord, you're it. I've nowhere else to turn."

Jesus says in John 12:24, "Truly, truly I say to you, unless a grain of wheat falls into the earth and dies, it remains by itself alone; but if it dies, it bears much fruit." Ironic isn't it? Here I am worrying about the prospect of dying, and yet in a sense, that's exactly what I need to do. When I made a covenant with God, I literally died to my own will and gave him my life. The only way out of this situation was through it, according to his will, his way and in his time.

I really do believe that nothing happens to us without first going through the Lord's hands. I didn't like it, but I knew God had allowed it. It could be that my resistance, my complaining and murmuring prolonged the process, but at least it hasn't been 40 years like the Israelites wandering in the desert. I used to read about their experiences, wondering why they never seemed to get it! I now have more compassion for them, as I've had my share of aimless wandering in this desert of mine. But the Promised Land is ahead, and I now know I'm going in the right direction. Today I can rejoice and give God praise for the trials and challenges he has allowed in my life and brought me through.

Take heart, beloved, because God is a good and loving Father. Every circumstance in your life can be offered to him, redeemed by him and transformed, completely changed for his glory. Isn't that awesome? He is able to take what was intended for destruction and evil and use it for good. Now, that is the God I serve and my prayer is that whatever is happening in your life right now, you will have the eyes of the spirit to see that God will cause everything to work for your good and his glory. Serving him is always worth the cost.

In Joel 2:25 the Lord promises,

> *I will restore to you the years that the swarming locust has eaten, the crawling locust, the consuming locust and the chewing locust, My great army which I sent among you; And My people shall never by put to shame. Then you shall know that I am in the midst of Israel and that I am the Lord your God and there is no other. My people shall never be put to shame.*

Perhaps your life has been ravaged by the enemy. But God is able to make all things new, bringing good from every situation. Welcome the fire of his spirit. Allow him to consume you until you are nothing in and of yourself and there is no resistance to his will for your life. Ask him to burn out all of your own sufficiency, your own power and pride. He is a God of new beginnings. Each time we encounter him, we have an opportunity to begin anew. In our brokenness of heart he comes in to establish restoration. Where there was sin he grants forgiveness. He gives joy for those in mourning, granting peace and power for the restless, fearful heart. He truly does make all things beautiful in his time.

**A Doctor's Report, or the Report of the Lord?**

I will never forget that day in February 1992 when I returned to the University of Washington medical clinic to hear the doctor's diagnosis. By that time I had undergone all the tests including blood tests, bone marrow biopsy, x-rays and urine tests. Then the hematologist, a specialist in the study of blood, sat down and proceeded to share his conclusions. In a calculating and detached way, he delivered the diagnosis, telling me that I had multiple myeloma, a terminal disease in stage three development. He told me that most people die from this type of cancer within three years. This physician could not have been more impersonal, clinical and lacking in empathy.

I felt myself go numb. Hearing that cancer diagnosis, I suddenly felt like I was receiving a physical blow. I felt angry and bewildered at his words. Then something inside of me rose up and said, "No! I am not going to receive this." He proceeded to explain that my best choice for a quality of life would be to agree to undergo a bone marrow transplant because they could give me five more years . . . if I were fortunate enough to live through that procedure. *Imagine that,* I thought. *Here he is acting like he knows exactly what the course of my life will be and when and how I will die. Does he think he's God?* How could this physician, a mere mortal, limited in power and authority, pronounce a death sentence over me? I can see how some people receive such a proclamation, which becomes a self-fulfilling prophecy. We all have a certain amount of respect for physicians, but perhaps we place them on a pedestal where they do not belong. They are not God. Patients must believe they can get well and overcome, no matter what the odds. Overcomers are those who push statistics aside and determine to beat the odds. As a hygienist and a member of the healthcare profession, I was familiar with the procedures of bone marrow transplants. To be honest, that procedure in itself scared me more than the disease. I couldn't believe that all these years of investigation and money spent on cancer research that this was the best treatment available. It seemed barbaric to me. Besides the transplant, the other option was to try to control the disease process, hoping that there might be a cure in the future.

There were no guarantees, of course. I didn't like either of the options.

I headed home, knowing I would need to deliver this news to my two sons Matthew and Joseph. By then my sons were 14 and 15 years old and certainly well aware of the possibility of the outcome of all the medical tests I'd been through. I dreaded having to go home and tell them the news. I knew I was so emotional that I would end up crying and exposing my vulnerability, and this was always uncomfortable for me. Anger again began to surface, as I anticipated delivering the news to them. I thought about the unfairness of life and the pain they had already experienced in their young lives.

It had been seven years since their father had decided to leave the marriage that ultimately resulted in divorce. And now this, another parent who was supposed to be the source of security and protection for children, diagnosed with terminal cancer. I was dreading having to deliver the news that day. My first response, after the numbing effect of this early shock, was anger toward God. "Lord," I said, "haven't we been through enough loss? Why this now? How could this be happening? You are all powerful, aren't you?" All kinds of wild, uncontrolled thoughts raced through my mind, trying to justify this situation, my life flashing before me, trying to recount all the sin I had committed in the past, thinking somehow this must have been my fault or that I had brought on this illness. Soon I was overwhelmed with my futile attempts to get an answer by trying to understand the age-old question, "Why?" The battleground was in my mind. The enemy of my soul was launching an all-out assault. In no time, my conflicting emotions were more than I could contain.

When I told my sons the news, we all sat down and had a good cry and hugged each other. There in the midst of the pain, disappointment and hurt the only thing I had to grasp onto was the hope that somehow God would take up my cause and intervene in this situation. But I knew that to be true in my mind, my heart was betraying me with all the emotional pain I was feeling. I could feel the Lord putting his arms around the three of us, and although I was still angry, he was there to comfort us. He understood our hurt and my fears.

Two of my friends, who were my prayer partners, were there to represent the arms and love of the Lord as they comforted us through this initial dreadful report. Our hearts were bonded together all the more in this very difficult time. Although my family of origin was not there for me, the Lord was going to show me how he would provide for us through his body, the church, the family of God.

Over the past twelve years since I had made a confession of faith, I discovered how God had provided a new family for me in the household of the believers. Little did I know that in the days, months and years ahead, God would reveal to me the genuine value of a healthy family, as well as the consequences of growing up in a toxic, dysfunctional family. Just then, as we cried and prayed, I knew I was grateful for the sincere and devoted friends that shared the love of Jesus and ministered to us in our time of need.

Over the next few days I struggled to make decisions, feeling pressured by the medical professionals who instilled in me a sense of urgency and fear. Since I knew no one else could tell me what to do, I had to come to a conclusion and create a plan. After I found a chance to settle down and get quiet, I knew I needed to seek the Lord and hear from him. I found a quiet place of solitude, opened my Bible and began to pray and seek the Lord through tears. I said: "Lord, if this is the time for me to come home, I do not want to fight your will. What I need is to know your perfect will in this situation." I never felt that my life was over at this point. But I was not going to be presumptuous, assuming I knew God's plans, which sometimes seemed to make no sense to me. As I waited on the Holy Spirit, I felt directed to read the passage from John 11, the passage about Lazarus. As I read the passage, the portion of scripture that seemed to be highlighted in yellow was John 11:4, where Jesus says, "This sickness will not end in death; no, it is for God's glory so that God's Son may be glorified through it." I had learned to listen to the Holy Spirit and get guidance, so I was confident as the Spirit put this scripture on my heart. I had a peace about the message and confirmation I was receiving. What I didn't realize is that I would cling to those words for many years until they would be manifest in my life.

During the weeks following that word and promise from God, I received confirmation of the scriptures from other people which helped strengthen my resolve, so I determined to take hold of that verse and do whatever I could to choose life. I made up my mind that there was no incurable disease, only incurable people. I could lose the war if I failed to get prepared for combat. The battle began.

Interestingly enough, as I looked back through my prayer journal I noted many times I had been praying for a healthy immune system. That thought struck me, since here I was, battling cancer which, in my understanding, was a failure of my immune system. As soon as I had my decision to battle the disease, my next decision was to determine how best to regain my health, designing a plan to halt this cancer that threatened to consume my life. I started my research, informing myself of both the disease and unconventional therapies that had been successful. In my mind, and in accordance to how I had been praying, I believed the best approach for treatment was to enhance and improve my own immune system.

I began to focus my research on immunotherapy. God created each of us with a miraculous body. With a healthy immune system, your body has an innate capacity to conquer disease and sickness. I wanted to give my body the best possible chance to do its job. So the search began. I am grateful for the information we have available today through the Internet. This way, I was not restricted to medical options in this country but literally had the world available to me. I began the quest for information and to establish a battle plan to address this challenge. Fortunately, I had always been interested in nutrition and good health, so I had a background and foundation for healthy living. It was not necessary to undergo a paradigm shift in my thinking. I had been seeing a naturopathic physician for years and was interested in alternative, complementary medicine. After gathering my information and looking for different modes of treatment, I consulted with my naturopath. One of my first decisions was to purchase a juicer so I could take advantage of the vitamins and minerals found in fresh raw juices. In this way, I began to increase nutritional support for my body. I also explored the concept of healing in spirit, soul and body. I began to understand that healing in the physical realm was not isolated from our whole being, not to the exclusion of the spirit and soul. I was beginning to be challenged in my thinking about what I believed to be true regarding health and illness. This was going to be quite a journey, and I had so much to learn.

Here is one of many journal entries from those days:

Dear Lord,
God, I feel so completely overwhelmed by all that is happening to me. I don't like this and I am angry about the situation. So many times I feel you have abandoned me and left me to struggle on my own. I know it doesn't help to ask why? It's not the right question but I thought I'd let you know it's how I feel right now. Totally without answers . . . lonely, frightened and struggling to believe and trust you . I know I am drawing upon my past experiences before I knew you but all those emotions are so strong and intense it's all I feel right now. When I can calm down my only comfort comes in reading your promises you have preserved for me in your word. I read them over and over because they help put my heart at rest and gain a hopeful perspective on this season of life. Help me please to trust you and lean upon you for all I need. You really are all I have. A part of me knows that somehow you will turn this situation around and use it for good both for me and for others. Lord, please give me the strength and courage to draw close to you and get through this trial. You have promised to direct and guide me and I am trusting you to do as you promise. It is only going to be by your spirit and strength dear Lord.
Your daughter,
Gretchen

**Personal reflections:**

1. If you have not kept a journal in the past, begin to record your life from this time on. The journal will prove to be therapeutic as you write, including all your emotional responses as well as a good reference for the healing process and a record of spiritual insights along the way. Pour your heart out before the Lord and watch the progress over the days and months ahead. You too will look back and see how faithful he has been throughout this season of life.

2. Meditate on these passages of scripture:

*Trust in the Lord with all your heart and lean not on your own understanding; in all your ways acknowledge him, and he will make your paths straight* (Proverbs 3:5–6).

*You will keep in perfect peace him whose mind is steadfast, because he trusts in you. Trust in the Lord forever, for the Lord, the Lord, is the Rock eternal* (Isaiah 26:3–4).

Seek out scriptures as God reveals his plan and purpose for your life. Begin to plant those promises in your heart, and commit them to memory.

3. Determine resources for information. Some examples:

National Cancer Institute
Alternative treatment options
Websites for cancer and therapies
Medical websites

# Inquire of the Lord

*Think of me as a fellow patient in the same hospital who, having been admitted a little earlier, could give some advice.* —C.S.Lewis

First, I decided I was going to live. I decided to make every effort to determine the best course of action that would prove healing for my entire being, including my spirit, soul and body. It is imperative to seek God's will, asking him what course of action to take each day. A terminal illness is only terminal because the medical profession does not have all the answers. Good news for those of us who know our God . . . he has all the answers!

Secondly, I evaluated all the treatment options I could gather, regarding their effects upon my entire being. I have included a chart to help you evaluate different treatment options and how they will influence or affect you. Fill out the chart as you research. Then evaluate after you have gathered all the information. The more informed you become, the better able you will be to make an informed decision. Take your time, resist fear and panic, and let God's peace and wisdom guide you.

As I did my research into the subject of cancer and disease generally, I came to discover a correlation between physical illness and the spiritual and emotional components of our being. The more I learned about my particular disease, the more I recognized the need for a miraculous intervention and God's grace. Humans did not have the answer! I was astounded to find out that no one had any answers to most of my questions, and medically there seemed to be very little hope. No one could tell me why I had this cancer. When I consulted people in the medical field, they seemed satisfied to treat symptoms without knowing the root cause. This bewildered me and was contrary to my frame of reference. After all, if we continue to treat symptoms and never address the root cause, how can we ever really be truly cured? I understood that God had created an intricate, complex wonderful body, including the immune system, which, given the opportunity, would overcome cancer and heal itself.

I have great respect for the medical profession. At the same time, however, I recognize there is a compelling divergence of opinions and philosophies within the community as to how to treat disease. The quest for me was to find that physician who was willing to work with me, understanding I was only going to take conservative, non-invasive therapy to help my own body do its job. It sounded quite reasonable to me. However, because of the medical establishment in this country and because of the influence of the pharmaceutical and insurance companies, any departure from standard protocol was not welcome, even when it was less costly, less invasive and potentially more effective.

There is a complex and often unclear assumption about what causes the cancer process. We all have cancer cells in our bodies. So why, and in what circumstances, does the cancer become opportunistic in some people? My journey led me to seek complementary medicine as a viable approach for healing. It included the options of conventional therapy, as well as a holistic approach to an individual, an approach that included the healing of body, soul and spirit. This integrative approach to health and wellness was the path and direction for me. I was determined to get to the root of my problem, physically, spiritually, mentally and emotionally. I know the Lord sees me as an integrated human being with a spirit, soul and body. One aspect of my being is not affected to the exclusion of the rest. This would only happen as God, in his grace, would reveal wisdom and knowledge along the way and keep me alive long enough to discover the path of healing. Here was a trial of my faith and a training ground with the opportunity to grow and to experience God's faithfulness to me. Every day, one day at a time, God would counsel and lead me in the way I would need to go.

Within the body of research about cancer, I kept reading about the influences of stress, including emotional trauma, negative thought processes, diet, environmental toxicity and more. The puzzle was becoming much more complex and yet it all made sense to me. I had an uncomfortable sense that in fact, my life history, including all my life experiences, may have had an influence and been a contributing factor in the development of this cancer. I was willing to address the issue, choosing to remain open-minded and tender hearted before the Lord.

Once I felt convinced about the approach I was going to take, I began to take action and put together a team of healthcare providers including the oncologist, the naturopathic physician, a nutritionist, an environmental specialist, an acupuncturist and a massage therapist. The team evolved over time as my health needs would arise and vary.

After consulting with my naturopathic physician I decided to go to a clinic in Mexico where I could receive treatment to boost my immune system and simultaneously help my body through a detoxification therapy. It was in Mexico that I heard about a physician in my own city who was an oncologist who, after years of practice had discovered far better success helping people overcome or live with cancer by incorporating a more holistic approach. If nothing else happened in Mexico, I reasoned, it was worth the trip to find this oncologist, and here he was in my backyard!

This physician was all I had hoped and prayed for in a clinician. He was a believer with a gracious attitude of humility and great respect for the human body as God had created it, recognizing the marvelous and miraculous capacity of the body to heal itself. He felt his job was to support and help the body do its job as designed by the Creator.

For the first time, after I had my visit with him I left his office with great hope and optimism and a belief that with God we could overcome this cancer battle. This was in sharp contrast to the other oncologists I had seen in the past. These encounters with the other physicians left me feeling hopeless, despairing and fearful because of their clinical, calculating attitudes. It always took me several days to overcome the encounters I had with these physicians, and then it always became a dreadful anticipation preparing for the next appointment.

When you are dealing with a serious, deadly enemy, you need all the support and encouragement possible, so I recommend drastic action where and when needed. I decided this was not good for me to anguish and fear my doctor's appointments so I fired those oncologists who had no faith and gratefully entrusted my care to the physician with excellent expertise as well as faith, hope and love. What a rare and gracious man of God. He fully appreciated and understood the importance of treating the whole person—spirit, soul and body—and gladly welcomed the team of other providers, including support for the spiritual and emotional components.

I caution anyone seeking medical treatment to evaluate the attitude and philosophy of any physician. Because medical science alone has tremendous limitations, it was essential that I have a physician who would embrace the value of the spiritual and emotional component in the healing process. By now I had done several things:

- I had done my research and felt confident about my ability to make an informed decision
- The decision I reached gave me a sense of peace
- A team of healthcare providers and support systems was in place
- I began a daily regimen of detoxification and nutritional restoration
- I have included the following chart to help you assess your different treatment options:

Identify problem/situation/circumstance:

## TREATMENT OPTIONS

|  | What is it called? | How does it work? | How effective is it? | What are positive aspects? | What are negative aspects? | Is this right for me? |
|---|---|---|---|---|---|---|
| Traditional **treatment** |  |  |  |  |  |  |
| Accepted **alternative** |  |  |  |  |  |  |
| Experimental **approach** |  |  |  |  |  |  |
| Other **strategies** |  |  |  |  |  |  |

### Self-Analysis (inventories)
**How does this affect my total being?**

| A. Personal |
|---|
| B. Emotional |
| C. Physical |
| D. Spiritual |

Specific prayer request:

Message or answer from God by scripture, another person or research:

Is it time to make a decision?

What decision?

Resources for more information:

Additional notes:

**Identify the Enemy and Learn the Tactics**

Research indicates that cancer, simply put, is a response of a cell whereby the cell becomes abnormal or rebellious and reproduces in an uncontrolled manner. It is a chronic, degenerative disease in which cells have become chemically altered mutations. As these cells begin to invade other healthy tissue, they cause damage. If the body's immune system fails to recognize these mutant cells, they will multiply and begin new colonies or tumors elsewhere in the body. There are many different types of cancers depending on the cell and location of the original mutant cell. In addition to these cells growing in an inordinate manner, they also function in a different way metabolically. Rather than using oxygen to metabolize energy as other cells do, they feed on the fermentation of glucose. As the tumors continue to grow, the body is starved of oxygen.

The cause of cancer is becoming clearer as time and research evolve. There does not seem to be one single issue or culprit but rather a combination of circumstances or contributing factors that predispose a person to cancer. Certain factors predispose a person to cancer. Here are some of those factors:

- genetic factors or family history

- nutritional deficiencies or imbalances
- chronic emotional stresses
- unresolved conflict
- environmental exposures, including industrial and automotive chemicals, cigarette smoke, heavy metal toxicity and radiation exposure
- improper diets: high fats and proteins, over-processed foods
- chemical exposure including pesticides, herbicides, solvents, formaldehyde
- poor drinking water due to hazardous chemical buildup
- excessive caffeine or alcohol
- endocrine imbalances (such as estrogen)

As you read the list above, you may be realizing that most cancer is a byproduct of our affluent, sophisticated Western lifestyles. The choices we have made as a nation—both corporately and as individuals—have contributed to our ill health and degenerative diseases, including cancers, heart disease, asthma, environmental illnesses and obesity. Patrick Quillin, Ph.D., reinforces this idea as he addresses our choices regarding nutrition:

> New estimates say that 90% of all cancer is environmentally caused and hence preventable. Environmental factors include foods, pollutants, sunlight, tobacco, etc. Of these environmental factors, nutrition is probably the most important. A conservative estimate states that 30–60 percent of all cancer is nutrition related. The U.S. has 500 percent more breast and colon cancer than other areas of the world, and much of this dubious distinction is caused by poor nutrition.[1]

By now you be overwhelmed by conflicted feelings as to how you got cancer in the first place. Don't despair. This information is meant to give you some guidance. You will see that there are several approaches to treating disease other than the conventional medical wisdom of surgery, chemotherapy and radiation, or what some have referred to as the "cut, poison and burn" methods.

As I began to understand that I did have some responsibility and perhaps contributed to my situation out of ignorance, I realized there were steps I could take to impact my healing process and give myself the best opportunity to recover. Most illnesses have a psychological component and a realization of one's own participation and responsibility in the disease process. This realization is entirely different from feeling blame and guilt.

I have taken part in the illness process and now I can take part in the recovery and restoration, which translates to empowerment. The miserable shortcoming of allopathic medicine is the failure to address the causes of cancer. This failure leaves a person feeling helpless and hopeless, as a cancer diagnosis becomes a deadly prognosis. Take heart, because there is much that can be done to strengthen your own body defenses and begin to help your immune system do its job.

Nutrition may well be your best medicine. In the long run it will work to correct the imbalances, deficiencies and cellular disturbances in the body, ultimately helping the body recover from illness as well as increasing vitality and strength for the days ahead. Many people have overcome their cancers, or at the very least are living with the disease, managing it much like any other non-fatal chronic illness. Many have successfully gone before you. You can take charge and do whatever it takes to live and be better than ever! You are not a powerless victim in the hands of physicians.

Doing whatever it takes to get well is time-consuming and demanding upon anyone, much less someone struggling with a life-threatening illness. There were plenty of times I wanted to give up, but I had too many good reasons to press forward and stay hopeful. I surrounded myself with people who would encourage me when I slipped in the dark hole of hopelessness, despair and self-pity.

Today I realize the valuable importance of community, particularly since we live in a society that esteems self-sufficiency and isolation. It became a humbling experience for me to continually ask for and receive help. I now had a prayer group, Bible study group, and cancer support group, in addition to the healthcare specialists. Not only was my body well cared for, but I also had the spiritual and emotional support I needed. I began to become encouraged as I read and researched more about alternative therapies and how people were successfully overcoming cancer using more humane therapies.

It was in my cancer support group one night that I heard about the impact of environmental toxins and the relationship of a toxic environment to cancer. Coincidentally, during that time, I had enrolled in a program to become a "master home environmentalist," which specializes in helping people identify potential sources of toxicity in the home and evaluate indoor air quality. I do marvel how God gets my attention. Time and again he confirms his will and direction to me.

More and more people have become chemically sensitive suffering from sick building syndrome and environmental illnesses. In the home environmentalist program, I learned that some patients don't respond to regular medical therapies because of internal burdens of multiple toxic compounds in their systems.

Environmental poisoning is no longer confined to poorly protected workers in toxic industries, but to all who breathe, eat, and drink, since these can now be toxic activities. Our environment has become flooded with chemicals that fill our air, water and food. It is no longer a question of whether we are carrying toxic loads. The question is, What effect do these chemicals have on our immune, endocrine and other bodily systems? What role do the chemicals play in one's health problems?

With this increased and widespread environmental contamination, we are facing increased rates of toxin-related cancers, neurological diseases, autoimmunity, reduced immune function, chronic fatigue, and fibromyalgia. Although I was aware of this information, somehow I had dismissed the possibility that I could contain toxins. After all, I had been routinely practicing a regimen that I thought would extract toxins from my system and keep me free of further toxic buildup. I had been on a program of raw juice therapy, colonic and enema therapy. Yet I was never sure about and had not confirmed what toxins I may have been carrying.

During our support group meeting that night, a woman shared about a cleansing and detoxification program she had recently completed with a physician who specialized in environmental disease. She was shocked to find out that there were heavy toxic loads in her system. I suddenly remembered when my doctor first diagnosed me. He had questioned me, in my interview, if I had been in any toxic environments such as living on a farm, involvement with certain hobbies, or exposure to solvents or chemicals. I actually had lived on a farm during periods of my life, both dairy and agricultural. As I listened to her, I became more receptive to pursuing more information and determining what chemical toxins might be in my body. It certainly made sense to me that such toxins could impact the health of a person adversely. I was skeptical, but at the same time I was determined to find out the answers. I would at least remain open-minded and research the subject.

I was referred to an environmental specialist. This was during a time when the myeloma disease process was very active and I was feeling desperate, not wanting to waste time and money. I told this physician about my feelings. After speaking with him and hearing about the expertise he had and the success of many cancer patients, I agreed to undergo testing for solvents, PCBs, pesticides, mercury and other heavy metal levels.

When I received the results back, I was stunned. I was full of toxins and I had a greater toxic load of solvents than any previous cancer patient! As a dental hygienist I had been exposed to mercury vapor in the office, I also had amalgam (mercury) restorations in my teeth. My mercury level was at very high toxic levels in addition to fairly significant levels of PCBs and pesticides. I was upset, but the environmental doctor smiled and said, "At least we have something to work with here. This could be why your immune system is so suppressed."

During that time, I also tested my natural killer cell activity, which is one measure of the immune system capacity. It was very low. Normal range was between 50 and 100, yet my level was only

17. My poor immune system was overwhelmed and not winning the battle. As a pattern during therapy this doctor had seen notable improvements in the immune system function after a person removed the toxins from their systems. I became convinced of the value of detoxifying my body and signed up for the battle. Battle it was. I don't think I've ever worked so hard and been so exhausted.

The detoxification program consisted of six weeks of an intensive regimen including thermal heat chamber, hydrotherapy, nutritional supplements and colonic therapy. Let me tell you, only the courageous and bold get through such a program. Not only would I need to survive the six weeks of intensive therapies, but also I would need to make some lifestyle adjustments. What choice did I have? I made the decision to move ahead, pay the price and believe this was another key in my journey to restoration in body, soul and spirit.

Perhaps it was because I had been in somewhat of a habit and discipline of cleansing and detoxification that I "hit the wall" early, as they say. This meant I entered a healing crisis, having symptoms of fever, nausea, weakness and general malaise. This is actually a positive response and indicates that the immune system is being challenged. So much for a positive response! Along with the physical crisis, I was experiencing emotional releases during that time. The Great Physician is always thorough when he heals. Not surprisingly, then, I was getting rid of some emotional toxins that had accumulated over the years. I was experiencing sorrow and grief over issues that were years old. I thought those griefs were behind me.

Someone once said that healing was like peeling an onion, one layer at a time. Each time one layer is removed, you get closer to the heart or core of the onion. Well, I felt like I was being stripped to the core all right. Being the type of person I am, I have always tended to stuff my emotions, and now I know that was not a healthy practice. God was stripping away many layers of grief and emotional sorrow that had been stored over a lifetime. The healing process was continuing on all fronts: physically, emotionally and spiritually.

---

[1] Patrick Quillin, Ph.D., R.D., Healing Nutrients (Chicago: Contemporary Books, 1987), page 127.

# The Detoxification Process

From a physical perspective, the thermal heat portion of the detoxification program forces the toxins out of the fat storage from the body reserves to the bloodstream, allowing these poisons to be excreted by the body. The hydrotherapy (hot and cold packs on the chest and back) stimulates blood flow and boosts the immune system. Finally, the colonic therapy helps to relieve the liver of chemical residue and clean the blood. Believe me, starting at 9:00 A.M. and ending the day at 6:00 P.M., Monday to Friday, was a rigorous schedule. I was exhausted at the end of those days. But whatever it would take to get well, I was going to do it, even if it meant crying my way through the whole ordeal. I did my share of complaining and crying, alright. After the six-week program, I needed to continue the regimen at home. To this day I have incorporated many aspects of the detoxification process as a lifestyle. The initial six-week inpatient treatment was very expensive, but I learned how to do all the procedures so I could adapt them into a home protocol.

Many toxins, including solvents, may take up to two years to exit the body. For some reason and it could be a genetic weakness, my body needs help in the detoxification process, so I believe this will be a lifestyle change for me. This protocol can be done at home, but I would always recommend you have medical supervision. Again, this is the kind of therapeutic, healing and treatment approach that made sense to me. Remove any offensive or noxious toxins or chemicals that may be causing or at the very least contributing to cellular destruction and creating an unhealthy internal terrain. Human beings are all unique. What might be medicine or food for one individual may be poison for another. For example, I am deathly allergic to penicillin, yet for others this drug has been a lifesaver. Any treatment therapy must be individualized for each person. Who really knows? What kind of research has been done evaluating the effects of these poisonous substances in our bodies? Our environment is loaded with toxins, and we are exposed every day. If we are not ridding our bodies efficiently, then what is the impact of these toxic loads as they accumulate?

Since we all have a certain toxic load, the issue is whether the toxins I have are causing a problem immunologically, compromising my ability to overcome cancer. Remember also that when you take medications, the body is forced to work harder to break down these chemicals and process them as well. Many chemotherapeutic drugs are harmful to healthy cells as well as the cancerous cells, adding to the toxic load in the system. Standard medical treatments of chemotherapy, radiation and surgery may retard the original growth of cancer or send it into remission, but they do nothing to restore the body's own protective systems or deal with the root cause. Cancer is a red flag that means something has gone wrong with the body's metabolic process. Any hope of winning the battle must include an aggressive program to restore healthy body function, change the body chemistry and restore balanced metabolic function.

The first stage of this process is detoxification, followed by restoration through optimum nutrition and diet. There are numerous resources available for a greater depth and understanding about the benefits of detoxification. I have included lists of information in the Appendix. See the Resource Section for recommended reading.

To induce your body to begin detoxification, proper nutrition is essential. When I was first diagnosed I had read about Dr. Max Gerson, a pioneer in the treatment of chronic illness, including cancer. Dr. Gerson's philosophy could be summed up in his statement: "There should be a treatment applied which will fulfill the task of totality in every respect, taking care of the functions of the whole body in all its different parts, thus restoring the harmony of all biological systems."[1] I started myself on the recommended protocol by Dr. Gerson, a process that included detoxification and rebuilding. Daily therapy included eight cups of raw juice, three or more coffee enemas and other medicinal and nutritional support. The raw juices containing live enzymes begin to clean out the body. Because the toxins begin to dump into the system the liver support is imperative. I added the sauna into my regimen after discovering the levels of chemical toxins and heavy metals, including mercury. As you may well imagine, without some sort of relief by means of enemas or colonic therapy, the toxins would recirculate and remain in the body. Not only does the liver filter all substances—including toxins—from the body, but it also activates enzymes that metabolize nutrients. These, in turn, nourish all the cells in the body. A healthy, well functioning liver is a must. Bile, produced in the liver, helps flush out the toxins from the body. If this process is slow or compromised, waste products and poisons can build up in the bloodstream.

Another source of ill health and compromised vitality is in the colon. I have heard it said that most illness begins in the colon. As the body toxins accumulate due in great part to the environmental toxins, our refined American diets and poor exercise, the colon can become encrusted with layers of thick rubbery buildup lining the walls of the intestine. Along with a cleansing protocol for the liver and gall bladder, I also included regular colonic therapy to cleanse the intestines. When you begin a detoxification routine, it is absolutely essential to stay ahead of the toxins with the coffee enemas to support the liver. In the beginning I was administering three coffee enemas per day. Dr. Linda Rector-Page, Ph.D. explained in her book *Healthy Healing,* "Coffee enemas have become standard in natural healing when liver and blood related cancers are present. Caffeine used in this way stimulates the liver and gallbladder to remove toxins, open bile ducts, encourage increased peristaltic action, and produce necessary enzyme activity for healthy red blood cell formation."[2]

Yes, it's true. My life centered on juicing eight cups of raw juice and preparing for coffee enemas. Whatever time I had left I was getting ready for the next round. Are you willing to do what it takes to get well? It's just for a season of life, so take heart: you will survive and feel better than ever! You will come to have a new, fond affection for coffee, quite different from the past. I've heard all the comments and jokes about coffee enemas. But remember, they can be life enhancing for many. Today, whenever I smell the wonderful aroma of coffee, my bowels start churning in anticipation. Remember Pavlov's dog? Same concept, I guess. Keep a sense of humor, and get started on your program. (See "Detoxification Techniques" in the Appendix.)

# Nutritional Supplementation

For whatever reason, the metabolic function of a person fighting cancer has been compromised. Because of this, the body is more often than not suffering some nutritional deficiencies. The liver is the most important organ in the body involved in detoxification. It is in the liver where toxic substances such as drugs, alcohol and environmental toxins are rendered less harmful to the system and are removed from the body. When the liver becomes compromised, the body does not properly metabolize some nutrients, so the body is starved of essential elements. Vitamin and mineral supplementation is imperative in the battle against cancer in order to support the body—in particular the liver—through the detoxification process. Later, this supplementation is necessary to rebuild and restore the body, reinforcing the body's capacity to fight off further disease.

There are no "quick fixes" when you choose to begin the process of restoring your health. There are no silver bullets when it comes to reversing the effects of years of developing a chronic degenerative disease. It takes time, energy and resources to get well. But when you consider the alternatives, you will be motivated.

The best source of vitamins, minerals and enzymes is from fresh, raw, organic foods. Current research would lead one to suspect that pesticides are carcinogenic and hormone-disruptive so until the evidence is conclusive I suggest you err on the side of caution. The 12 most contaminated fruits and vegetables are strawberries, bell peppers, spinach, cherries, peaches, Mexican cantaloupe, celery, apples, apricots and green beans. Find a good health food store. You will find this will become familiar territory.

Because of the compromised metabolic problems with cancer patients, there is a need to supplement your diet with additional nutritional support. Yes, you may have expensive urine for a while, but at least you will be supplying your system with all it needs. Dr. Harold W. Harper has written: "Degenerative diseases are not caused by viruses, bacteria, or parasites, but by the body's inadequate metabolic response to a condition in which the cells of the body are being slowly poisoned by too many of the wrong things or not enough of the right things at the right time."[3] I have provided a chart for you, listing the bare essentials of my nutritional program. Over the years the list has varied, depending upon circumstances, but those I have included are essential. Your nutritionist or naturopathic physician will be the best person to design a nutritional support program to meet your individual needs. Additionally, certain herbal, homeopathic and other supplements may be beneficial for you.

## Table of Supplements and Nutritional Support

| VITAMIN/SUPPLEMENT/ NUTRIENT | FUNCTION/SUPPORT |
|---|---|
| **Vitamin A:** fat soluble, requires fats and zinc, minerals, enzymes for absorption; heat stable; unstable to air; UV light destroys it. | Develops strong bones, immune system with increased resistance. Counteracts night blindness, weak eyesight. Reverses pre-malignant changes in tissue. |
| **Beta-Carotene:** vitamin A precursor, converting to vitamin A in the liver. | Anti-infective and anti-oxidant for immune health. Protects against environmental toxins. A key in preventing some cancers and supporting anti-tumor immunity. |
| **B-Complex Vitamins:** water-soluble, should be used together for broad spectrum activity. | Essential for all functions. |
| **Vitamin B1-Thiamine:** unstable to ultraviolet; destroyed by boiling in acidic solution, heat. | Beneficial effects on nervous system and mental attitude. Enhances immune response, blood building, carbohydrate metabolism, learning ability. Promotes growth; improves resistance to infection. |
| **Vitamin B2-Riboflavin:** water-soluble; unstable to UV; destroyed by alkalines. | Promotes antibody and red blood cell formation. Aids iron assimilation and protein metabolism; healthy skin and digestive tract; vision. |

| | |
|---|---|
| **Vitamin B3-Niacin:** water-soluble; stable in heat. | Promotes circulation; hormone production; growth; HCl production; metabolism; respiration. |
| **Vitamin B5-Pantothenic acid:** water-soluble; unstable in heat; destroyed by acid/alkaline | Promotes antibody formation; carbohydrate metabolism; growth stimulation; healthy skin and nerves. Maintains blood sugar level. Stimulates adrenals. |
| **Vitamin B6 –Pyridoxine:** water-soluble; stable in heat; unstable in light. | Promotes antibody formation. Controls levels of magnesium in blood and tissues. Aids digestion. Maintains sodium potassium balance; metabolism of fats. |
| **Vitamin B12-Cyanocobalamin:** water-soluble | Helps with appetite; blood cell formation; cell longevity; normal metabolism of nerve tissue; protein; fat and carbohydrate metabolism, glandular and nervous system. |
| **Vitamin B15-Pangamic Acid:** water-soluble | Cell oxidation and respiration. Stimulates glucose, fat, protein metabolism, glandular and nervous system. |
| **Biotin-Vitamin H:** water-soluble; stable in heat; inactivated by oxidation; synthesized by intestinal bacteria. | Necessary for metabolism of amino acids and essential fatty acids and in formation of antibodies; enhanced immune response in Candida Albicans. |
| **Choline-Lipotropic and B complex family** | Helps emulsify fats. Brain nutrient and neurotransmitter; aids in memory and learning. Health of liver, kidney; prevents gallstones. |

| | |
|---|---|
| **Folic Acid-folacin, B complex family:** water-soluble, heat and light sensitive | Necessary for synthesis of DNA, enzyme efficiency and blood formation. Prevents anemia, helps control leukemia and pernicious anemia. HCL production; protein metabolism. |
| **Inositol:** water-soluble | Helps brain cell nutrition; fat metabolism; growth and survival of cells in bone marrow, eye and intestine. Promotes hair health. Reduces blood cholesterol. Protects liver, kidney and heart. |
| **PABA (a B- complex member):** water-soluble | Contains sun-screening properties, used in treating vitiligo, successful with molasses, pantothenic acid, and folic acid in restoring lost hair color; protein metabolism. Helps in formation of folic acid. |
| **Vitamin C-Ascorbic Acid:** water-soluble; stable to heat; destroyed by oxygen, U.V., copper and iron cooking vessels, pasteurization, canning, insecticides. | Strengthens and maintains immune system; blood vessel health. Helps reduce cancer risk; collagen production. Increases resistance to infection. Promotes proper bone and tooth formation; red blood cell formation. |
| **Bioflavonoids (part of C complex):** water-soluble. | Helps prevent arteries from hardening. Strengthens blood vessel, capillary and vein. Lowers cholesterol levels. Stimulates bile production, anti-microbial against infections. Reduces cataract formation. |

| | |
|---|---|
| **Vitamin D (sunlight vitamin):** fat soluble | With vitamin A, uses calcium and phosphorus in building bone structure and healthy teeth. Helps protect against colon cancer. |
| **Vitamin E:** fat soluble anti-oxidant | Simulates immune system; anticoagulant and vasodilator against blood clots and heart disease. Alleviates fatigue. Works with selenium to neutralize free radicals against the effects of aging and cancer. |
| **Vitamin K:** fat soluble | Necessary for blood clotting; heals broken blood vessels in eyes. Aids in arresting bone loss; anti-parasitic for intestinal worms. |
| **Vitamin P- Bioflavonoids:** water-soluble, occurs with vitamin C with similar properties. | Alters permeability of capillaries; increases resistance to colds and flu; maintains healthy connective tissue and blood vessel walls. |
| **Minerals:** essential to proper body function. Work in conjunction with vitamins to provide building blocks. | Many minerals have been identified as efficacious in fighting cancer. (I always take extra selenium, magnesium, calcium, and zinc.) |
| **Amino Acids:** anti-oxidant; building blocks of protein in the body. | Cleans the blood of toxins and effects of drug therapy. (I take extra glutathione for detoxification.) |

| | |
|---|---|
| **Essential Fatty Acids-EPA-DHA, Omega 3, Omega 6** | Known to stimulate production of prostacyclin, which help to purge body of cancer growths; also known to stimulate the immune system; has cardiovascular benefits. |
| **Colon Fiber Cleanse** | Bentonite clay and psyllium husks in combination provide cleansing of the colon for removal of toxins, metals, drugs; helps promote friendly intestinal bacteria and retention of B-complex vitamins. |
| **Green Drinks:** wheatgrass juice, raw green vegetables from organic sources, barley green drinks, kelp, algae, chlorella. | Super food for the body. Includes amino acids, chlorophyll, minerals, enzymes, vitamin A, beta-carotene, calcium, iron, potassium. Blood builders. |
| **Raw Glandular Extracts:** provide nutrients that aid the reproduction of cells for the particular organ or gland. | Desiccated liver and adrenal extract were an essential adjunct for my recovery. Determine the organs that are insufficient and augment with glandular therapy. |
| **Pancreatic Enzymes** | Normally produced by the liver to help with food digestion. Also known to attack the cell wall of cancer cells, allowing the immune system the capacity to destroy them. |
| **Herbal Therapy** | Chinese herbs and other herbal therapies are becoming recognized for their healing capacity. |

| | |
|---|---|
| **Intra-Rectal Nutrients:** the most profound and innovative part of the detox and restoration of the body. Formulated by Allergy Research Group/ Nutricology: 800-545-9960<br><br>15 grams of vitamin C from a corn source<br>30 MEQ or 15 ml or magnesium chloride<br>2 ml of trace mineral<br>2 grams of taurine<br>600 mg glutathione<br>2 ml of B complex, incl. 2 ml of B-12 | Formally, over the years I have had intravenous vitamin drips which were never covered by insurance. Here is a product, developed by this company, which is in some ways preferable to IV nutrients and far less expensive. They have a booklet with instructions and suggestions. |

# Spiritual Healing

*I pray that you may enjoy good health and that all may go well with you, even as your soul is getting along well.* —3 John 2

One of the first things I did after I had been diagnosed with multiple myeloma was to seek out spiritual help and counsel. I was convinced that sin in a person's life could be causing a physical illness. I had known of a couple whose ministry it was to pray for the sick. I made an appointment with them, believing it was a biblical principle to seek prayer and be willing to address any spiritual malady as well as physical challenges.

When I first met this couple I was encouraged and felt safe sensing the love and compassion of Jesus they offered me. They proceeded to ask me to give a lengthy inventory of all my life events from the history of my family, including previous generations, to the present day circumstances. In the process of the interview, it became apparent to them and to me that I had suffered significant trauma throughout my life. This trauma included the death of my father at a young, vulnerable age, emotional abandonment by an alcoholic mother, miscarriages, divorce and now a life-threatening illness.

By this time, knowing what I did about illness and disease, I could look back and realize the impact of these circumstances on my life: my spiritual, emotional and physical well-being.

This couple prayed for me, starting in a chronological order and always ministering the love of Jesus to these areas of brokenness in my soul. I had been aware of many of the issues and had thought I had dealt with them. But I was again amazed at the emotional grief still residing in my soul. They prayed the Lord would reveal which issues should be dealt with, and in what order. This was a spiritual, emotional and mental inventory. I was feeling like a trout, just hooked and filleted open to reveal everything on the inside.

This was going to be a painfully transparent procedure. But I was willing to do whatever it would take to be well and restored. My life history continued to unfold before them. There have been many others who have graciously blessed me with the love of Jesus Christ, the love that is able to bring restoration and healing.

I always figured I had grown up in a normal home. But I gradually realized things were not normal, considering the impact of my father's death when I was nine years old. On that day, as the eldest of three daughters, I instantly became what seemed like an adult. Suddenly, life was different; I felt vulnerable and lost a certain sense of innocence. My mother was left widowed with three little girls, and when she became a real estate agent in order to support us, I felt a great sense of responsibility to care for my younger sisters. I carried that burden for many years. Life had changed dramatically.

In all my years of growing up my mother always made sure we all attended church on Sundays. My maternal grandmother was a Sunday school teacher, and she left a perpetual impression on her children. I know my grandmother was a godly woman who faithfully prayed for her family, including her grandchildren.

All the miracles started when I made a decision one day to ask the Lord Jesus Christ to come into my life and be lord of my life. It was a simple prayer that changed the course of my entire life.

It all began when, as a young bride, life before me seemed wonderfully optimistic and limitless. As a couple, we had enjoyed financial prosperity and good health, and our dreams and goals were being realized. Here we were at relatively young ages with two sons, a lovely home in suburbia and two Mercedes in the garage. Life only seemed to get better after the birth of each of our sons. Joy upon joy.

Although I had not been in an intimate relationship with the Lord, it was important to me, even then, to give my sons names having biblical significance. Matthew means "a gift from God," and Joseph means "increasing faithfulness." Providentially, and certainly by no mere coincidence, these young men have lived up to their prophetic names. When the boys were ready for preschool, they were enrolled in a Christian program. Again I had sensed a need to maintain consistency with my roots and heritage, treasuring the pleasant memories I had of those times in church and Sunday school. Once the boys were in preschool, however, I felt empty, unfulfilled, and happiness seemed to elude me. Like the singer I asked myself, "Is that all there is?" Although I was not in a boring routine and had attained my dreams and goals, I was dissatisfied. I was not in the habit of praying, but in desperation I said, "God, if you're there, I think I need to know you."

God was quick to answer my cry. Within a week, a friend from church invited me to a Bible study group for women called Bible Study Fellowship (BSF). This occurred near the beginning of the school year. I would take my sons to preschool and then head to church for BSF on Wednesdays. That first year in BSF was the study of the book of John. I was resistant yet inquisitive, as I challenged what I was learning. A breakthrough came for me when I read and understood that God loved me and was willing to lay down his life for me. How could this be, so great a love, that Jesus would give his life for me? The words of the life of Christ came to life, and I was overcome with his great love for me. I was overwhelmed with the love of Jesus.

One day I came to the scripture in Matthew 16:15–16, where Jesus asks his disciples,

> *"Who do people say the Son of Man is?" They replied, "Some say John the Baptist; others say Elijah, and still others, Jeremiah or one of the prophets." "But what about you?" he asked, "Who do you say I am?" Simon Peter answered, "You are the Christ, the Son of the living God."*

Like Peter, I came to the reality of needing to decide just who this Jesus is. It was love that he had for me, love that drove him to die a painful, humiliating death to take my place as payment for sin. He captured my heart that day and I love him more and more all the time. Like Peter, I came to know who this Jesus was. I am eternally grateful that he revealed himself to me and has given me new life. Before knowing my creator, life had become obscure and purposeless. It was like seeing life in black and white, knowing something is missing. Knowing the love of other human beings was different than God's love. Only God knows all the secret thoughts and intentions of my heart. Beyond my comprehension, he loves me in spite of all the faults and sins. The book of 1 Corinthians describes God's kind of love, which is

> . . . *patient and kind. It does not envy, it does not boast, it is not proud. It is not rude, it is not self-seeking, it is not easily angered, it keeps no record of wrongs. Love does not delight in evil but rejoices with the truth. It always protects, always trusts, always hopes, always perseveres. Love never fails.*

No human has the capacity to love to the depth and completeness of my Lord. I was always looking for what could truly satisfy my soul. I made the decision to turn my life over to him and allow him to be Lord of my life as well. I came to know my value and identity as a person because of him. His presence was like cool water seeping into the cracks of a parched desert. Suddenly, life began to spring forth because of the living water of the Holy Spirit. For the first time I felt an unbridled sense of hope and joy about being alive.

It is comforting and reassuring to know that God loves me and is orchestrating my life according to his plans, which are always for my best and for his glory. Prayer would become more essential in my life than I had ever known it to be before. After all, it really is a conversation with my loving heavenly father.

Here is another journal entry of mine:

Dear Father,
I am in awe of your love and mercy to me. How you found me and called me to yourself with such a persistent love. You are life itself and I cannot imagine living in this world apart from you. Thank you so much for saving me and making me your child. Your love is more than I can contain at times and

it's that love that satisfies me to the depths of my being. You purchased my life on the cross, exchanging my shame, bondage and guilt for your identity and freedom and now I give you complete control over my life. I'm not sure what it all means but I can trust you to guide me, provide for me and work all the circumstances in my life for my best. While I'm here on earth you will always be working to conform me to your dear son's image and extend the love you have given to me to others. In faith I say, "Have your way and cause your will to be done." I may not like it all the time but please stay with me and help me work through this process. I always want to remain humble before you and learn to trust you more all the days of my life. What a magnificent glorious love you have shown to me. All I really have to offer you is myself. I am eternally grateful and give you my life, trusting you to bring your purposes and plans to pass. I am eternally grateful and always yours . . . Gretchen

**Personal Reflections:**

1. *"For I know the plans I have for you," declares the Lord, "plans to prosper you and not to harm you, plans to give you a hope and a future."* —Jeremiah 29:11.

   Rewrite the above verse, substituting your own name for "you."

2. Talk to God and tell him how you are feeling and what you are thinking. Write him a letter, and in his own intimate way he will answer.

3. What hopes and dreams of your life have been realized?

4. What hopes and dreams have been dashed?

5. Take time to reflect over your life. Bring yourself before the Lord with a new and fresh willingness to allow him to search you and bring healing, deliverance and freedom to the deep levels of your soul. As you allow him to bring to light every area of your life, begin to journal any illumination from the word and any insight he may show you about yourself. God may reveal circumstances, situations, attitudes or influences that he wants to address to bring healing. I believe it is always productive and fruitful to periodically take our personal inventory.

More scriptures for your meditation times:

**Psalm 19:12** *Who can discern his errors? Forgive my hidden faults. Keep your servant also from willful sins; may they not rule over me. Then will I be blameless, innocent of great transgression.*

**Psalm 51** See entire psalm.

**Psalm 79:8–9** *Do not hold against us the sins of the fathers; may your mercy come quickly to meet us, for we are in desperate need.*

**Psalm 139** See entire psalm.

# Working Out My Salvation . . . One Day at a Time

*There is a kind of waiting you teach us—the art of not knowing.* —William Stafford, poet

My life had changed dramatically that day with a simple prayer, and it has not been the same since. The couple who had ministered to me early on in the diagnosis told me they would soon be leaving for the mission field, stationed in the outer parts of Siberia. That was a long way to go for prayer, so I had to have confidence that God would continue to send the people who would pray for me and encourage me along the path of healing.

I had learned some principles from them, and now I would continue to seek the Lord and trust him to continue my healing. I began to surround myself with faith-filled people who would continue to remind me of God's promises, pray for me and minister to both my soul and spirit. Scripture indicates that while here on earth we are to be working out our salvation every day.

Paul says in Philippians 2:12–13:

*Therefore, my dear friends, as you have always obeyed—not only in my presence, but now much more in my absence—continue to work out your salvation with fear and trembling,*

> *for it is God who works in you to will and to act according to his good purpose.*

The definition of that term *salvation* implies a wholeness, deliverance and completeness. Clearly, I have not reached perfection and do not have all truth. Working out that salvation is a lifelong process. It made sense to me that as I was choosing a physician to help with the physical healing that it would be equally important to choose people to minister to my soul and spirit. From the beginning I made the decision to always seek the Lord's counsel, to "inquire of the Lord" as I made decisions about which direction to go. All along the way God has been faithful to provide me with people of excellent character and wisdom. I submitted myself to counsel and to prayer, and through this journey some things began to come to light.

The Holy Spirit is ruthless in his pursuit to bring us to a place of freedom, deliverance and restoration. The Lord kept bringing me face to face with hindrances, sins and shortcomings that would cause me to experience the consequences of this bondage if I chose not to address them.

Hebrews 12:1 encourages us to

> *lay aside every encumbrance and the sin which so easily entangles us, and let us run with endurance the race that was set before us, fixing our eyes on Jesus the author and perfecter of faith, who for the joy set before him endured the cross, despising the shame, and has sat down at the right hand of the throne of God.*

I was attempting to run the race, all right, and now I had run headfirst into a brick wall. It may have stopped me temporarily, but walls are not a problem for God. After my experience in BSF, I moved into leadership with a new group of women, a ministry with an emphasis on Bible study and greater opportunity for fellowship and ministry.

It was during this time, after about three years of knowing Jesus personally, that I was undergoing conflict and trouble in my marriage, experiencing a painful time of separation, which eventually led to divorce. My friends from my Bible study group had invited me to a worship seminar one weekend with 1500 believers. Because I was hungering for God, I chased after every opportunity to gather in his presence and worship.

Shortly after I had come to a personal relationship with the Lord, he placed me in a church that I would describe as God's emergency room. Previously, I had been brought up in the mainline denominational churches and was unfamiliar with the more charismatic churches and the manifestation and work of the Holy Spirit. Feeling grief and pain from the marital conflict and the shame associated with it, I had cried out for a church where I would know his love, acceptance and forgiveness.

Week after week God touched me, and more and more I was strengthened. There was a sweet liberty of the spirit in this place, and I am grateful for the ministry of this body as they loved me with the love of Jesus and allowed the Holy Spirit to begin to heal my broken heart. God was beginning to expose those hindrances and sins in my life that were undermining the race he had called me to.

One of those dark areas in my life had to do with the impact of the alcoholism in my family of origin and now in my marriage. As I began dealing with the issues of my past and in particular, the alcoholism of the loved ones in my life, my husband decided to leave the marriage, since I was changing and would not continue to enable drinking behaviors.

The alcoholics in my life were people who managed their lives with some competency and were not people who had lost everything to the demon of alcohol addiction. My understanding of an alcoholic had been someone who had lost it all and was a street-gutter drunk. Both my mother's side of the family and my father's side of the family were plagued with members who struggled with alcohol addiction, but it was all very much a secret and no one wanted to admit that there was a problem.

Because of this, I had been steeped in a lifestyle of enabling the alcoholics in my life. I had a problem, and it was diagnosed as codependency. I was performing for others and all the time destroying the person I was born to be, having lost a sense of my own identity. Now I was confronted with living a lifestyle that was opposed to the family system, and when I decided to be truthful about all the family secrets I became a threat to my loved ones.

Truth often carries with it consequences, and I needed to decide what path to take. More than anything I wanted to be a truthful person, and I certainly wanted to give my sons the gift of freedom from the addiction cycle, so I made the decision to become informed about addiction and get counseling to change my behaviors as a codependent.

Sadly, the changes I chose were causing a wedge between my husband and me, because he was not prepared to change. He chose to maintain his lifestyle and leave the marriage. My choices also caused a chasm with my family of origin, because all my loved ones were caught in the addiction cycle at some level. My honesty and confrontation was not a welcome intrusion for the family system. I had violated the silent, unwritten rules and exposed the truth.

I was at a crossroads: would I choose to go on with Jesus, or maintain the status quo? With God I could overcome this obstacle. I chose to move forward. I must tell you, everything inside of me conflicted with what I knew to be the truth now. I could never have pursued the truth, had God not given me the courage.

As I was grieving over the loss of my husband and the marriage, I discovered I was also grieving for my father. This was all confusing and surprising to me and did not seem to make sense. After all, my father had died 21 years ago. What was happening?

All during this time I was in the word of God, with an insatiable desire to feed upon the promises. I had no one else to turn to for support, because my family was feeling threatened by my faith. I had a burning hunger and thirst for more of God. As I read the Bible and kept seeking his will and answers to my dilemma, God impressed the scripture from Ephesians 4:26–27 upon my heart: "In your anger do not sin, do not let the sun set on your wrath, lest you give Satan a foothold."

In other words, when I was angry, full of wrath, exasperation, fury or indignation I was not to hold onto it long and certainly not after sunset or the day ended. Doing otherwise would give the devil an opportunity. Now I was not clear about all the implications of this scripture, but I kept asking God for clarification and asked for help in dealing with anger. Anger wasn't wrong, but I needed to deal with it in a healthy way. My habit in the past was to deny the anger and stuff it down, because I had learned early on in my home that anger was not acceptable. Right then and there, I had good reasons to be angry, but I sure didn't want to be sinning.

There was so much confusion about all that God wanted to teach me. He was beginning to teach me healthy ways of handling painful circumstances and dealing with emotions honestly and openly before him. For someone who had spent a lifetime learning to deny and bury feelings, suddenly I was feeling exposed and vulnerable as God put his finger on these issues of my heart.

It was during this time that I attended the seminar with my friends. I had never experienced anything like what transpired during that weekend. It was a powerful time with so many believers gathered together, seeking God and worshipping in unity. Have you ever noticed how the presence of God is greater during a corporate gathering? It was a secure, loving atmosphere and must have been a sweet aroma and fragrance before the Lord at the throne of grace . . . so much so that he showed up.

I was unaccustomed to seeing the spirit of God freely moving among his people, touching lives and providing for the needs of every heart. Some people were crying, others were experiencing a deep peace and some were undergoing deliverance.

Admittedly, I was reticent at first. But as I saw miracle after miracle, people being set free, healed physically, delivered from spiritual oppression and freed from addictive habits, I was in awe of God once more. It reminded me of reading the book of Acts and the ministry of the apostolic church. Jesus was still moving among his people, every bit alive today as then.

At one point in the meeting there was an invitation to receive a fresh in-filling of the Holy Spirit. I figured that was a worthy, safe request, and the Lord knew I was thirsting for more of him. So, with courage, I went forward for prayer. As I stood before the Lord, ready to receive from him, I started crying. Believers gathered around me and began to lay hands on me and pray. The Lord began to reveal to me some unresolved issues connected with my father's death. I felt like a little child all over again, sobbing uncontrollably. Layer after layer of stored-up grief flowed from my innermost parts. The Lord gave me an impression of the day my father had died when I was nine years old. Suddenly, I was aware that I had never released my father and had never been allowed to grieve his death and let him go. The Lord was present now, and I was surrounded by loving people. After 20 years it was safe and acceptable to let out the grief.

It had all happened many years ago. I came home from school one day, confronted by many people in my home: strangers, relatives and friends. I was told that my father had been hospitalized with a severe problem and that he might not live. I went numb. Three days later, my father died of a cerebral vascular accident. As I remembered the sequence of the events of that day, I could see myself the night my father died: I was in my childhood bedroom alone, terrified and angry that my father had died and abandoned me. Then, just as if time had not passed, right there in that room I could sense Jesus' loving presence. I knew I could let go of my dad, forgive him for leaving and accept my heavenly father's love.

As a child growing up in an alcoholic, toxic family, I never was comforted or nurtured during this loss. All I could do to survive was to suppress all those painful, unacceptable emotions. The enemy of our souls does not play fair, and because I held this suppressed anger in my heart these years, I had given him a foothold in my life.

Suddenly the words of the passage from Ephesians flooded over my mind and heart, and I knew instantly what the Lord was showing me: I needed to let the anger go, not bottle it inside me. Indeed, I had been angry at the loss of my father and never having worked through the grief process and resolved the anger. In this way, I had given Satan a foothold. But that night, in his grace and mercy God delivered me from the bondage of spiritual oppression, including self destruction, rage, fear, bitterness, and torment. These oppressive spirits had access to my life because of an open door that resulted from an emotional trauma. I suffered the consequences of this oppression because I had hidden and suppressed the emotions.

After that deliverance, just like in the book of Acts, the presence of the Lord was so powerful and consuming, having come into my being and filled those previously occupied places, that I felt and appeared drunk in the spirit. I felt filled with his presence and joy, because he had replaced the weight of depression, guilt and shame. As the Lord drove out these enemies of my soul, I had a greater sense of his presence within. For several months following this deliverance, I often found myself weeping, not with tears of pain or grief or sorrow, but with tears of gratitude and thanksgiving. The fact that my heavenly father would intervene in such a powerful, lifesaving, life-changing way was more than my heart could contain from time to time.

The Bible warns about a bitter root in the book of Hebrews. Interestingly, that scripture had been part of my devotions the week before that deliverance. Hebrews 12:15: "See to it that no one misses the grace of God and that no bitter root grows up to cause trouble and defile many."

As I had suppressed all that anger and rage, it eventually became a root of bitterness that had given a foothold to the enemy of my soul. All these years I had silenced and suppressed this anger over my father's death to the point that I no longer was even aware of it. As I got in touch with that anger, though, I experienced a very forceful and powerful release because there was a great deal of energy connected to the anger and rage in my soul. I believe it was like a poison to my physical system, because as that rage was released I smelled a noxious burning sulfur smell. I believe God allowed me to sense how utterly destructive and deadly this rage had been to my body. After that emotional release, I felt a sense of freedom and strength return to body. On that occasion God healed me spiritually from the oppression of the enemy, healing my heart from the burden of grief I had carried. I know my body enjoyed a new sense of freedom and energy as a result. The Lord had promised me in Exodus that indeed he was going to drive the enemy out of my life, but it would not be all at once, but a process of deliverance. As the Lord tells the Israelites in Exodus 23:29,

> But I will not drive out (your enemies) in a single year, because the land would become desolate and the wild animals too numerous for you.

Just as the Lord took care of the enemies of the Israelites, he was going to deliver me from my enemies.

Prayer was effective in revealing further hidden faults or sins of mine. Although I was unaware of what was in my heart, the Lord knew very well. My part was to continue to humble myself, ask for prayer and maintain an attitude of humility as God continued with the healing process. The word from 1 Peter 5:6–11 was a continual encouragement to me:

> Humble yourselves, therefore, under God's mighty hand, that he may lift you up in due time . . . be self-controlled and alert. Your enemy the devil prowls around like a roaring lion looking for someone to devour. Resist him, standing firm in the faith . . . and the God of all grace, who called you to his eternal glory in Christ, after you have suffered a little while, will himself restore you and make you strong, firm and steadfast.

This new attitude of prayer was to be a transforming kind. I made a decision that I would get myself in front of God every chance I could and be transformed by his power and presence.

I wanted more of God, with no openings that would leave me vulnerable to the attacks from the enemy. I think God likes it when we diligently and persistently pursue him. He has always met me when I have such an attitude.

On another occasion, a man came to town who has been used of God powerfully in the area of evangelism in developing countries. He also has the gift of healing. Mahesh Chavda, originally from a Hindu family, had come to know the Lord at age 16 through missionaries to India. Moving and ministering in the anointing of the spirit of God does not come without cost. Mahesh is one of those brothers who has paid the price, by giving himself to a lifestyle of prayer and fasting, disciplines which were instilled in him from childhood.

I went to hear Mahesh preach and minister. After a time of Bible teaching, which created an atmosphere of faith, Mahesh moved into a time of ministry and called out various infirmities, diseases and sicknesses. I went forward when he called out cancer. When my turn came for prayer, Mahesh gently placed his hand beside my head and said, "By the authority of the Lord Jesus Christ I command the power of the sins of the forefathers to be broken, and I command a spirit of death and cancer to come out."

Once again, in my physical body I felt a manifestation of a release and breaking of power as my body experienced another level of freedom. Then I remembered the scripture from Genesis 20:5, where the Lord speaks of sin passing through the generations:

> *I the Lord your God am a jealous God, punishing the children for the sin of the fathers to the third and fourth generation of those who hate me, but showing love to thousands who love me and keep my commandments.*

Now I knew that my father's side of the family was rebellious and ungodly, so it was no surprise to me when this word was prayed over me and at the name of Jesus and by his power that curse was broken. Did I really understand the consequences of sin, my own and that of my forefathers, and how they impacted future generations? Another enemy driven out.

Could this spiritual and emotional healing be part of the healing of my physical body? There seemed to be a pattern emerging before me. First I was healed spiritually by being born anew by the spirit of God, by coming into right relationship with him. Then the Lord began healing my heart and soul. As my heart is being healed, my emotions are becoming free, which seems to have a positive healing effect upon my body. The emotions of fear, anger, bitterness, grief and depression all have had a detrimental effect upon my body. Proverbs 17:22 says, "A cheerful heart is good medicine, but a crushed spirit dries up the bones." With all these circumstances in my life I had indeed experienced considerable grief and a crushed spirit. Could there be a direct relationship between the thoughts of my mind, the emotions in my heart and the health of my physical body? Something to consider.

My spiritual support over the years has consisted of my church family and pastor, my prayer group and close friends who all believed in the power of prayer and believed that God heals today. When it came to whom I asked to pray for me, I was selective, after having had some painful experiences along the way.

It's important to recognize God's gifts in people and their callings. For instance, I would not advise a person with a strong administrative calling to lead in prayer ministry. Compassion, love and patience are requirements for the ministry of healing. Thankfully, I had a number of close friends who were intercessors, who had many years of experience ministering to people in the area of healing. You will find people who have a particular gift in this area of prayer.

I found that through prayer, God was beginning to heal the areas of my emotions, and through the Word of God my mind was being transformed and renewed to faith in the promises of God. Faith is nurtured and grown by hearing the Word of God.

I experienced many moments when I doubted God's willingness and his ability to take care of me in my situation. I asked the Lord to search my heart and continue to reveal any willful or hidden sins. Those sins of unforgiveness, anger, bitterness, resentment and more which would give the enemy of my soul a foothold, allowing access to my life. My desire was to submit myself to the purifying, cleansing work of the Holy Spirit and make sure there was no open door in the form of sin in my heart. Hebrews 4:12 says,

> *The word of God is living and active, sharper than any double-edged sword, it penetrates even to dividing soul and spirit, joints and marrow; it judges the thoughts and attitudes of the heart. Nothing in all creation is hidden from God's sight.*

I shudder whenever I read this passage, in anticipation of what might be known about me. Nothing is hidden from God's sight! But no matter what is in my heart, God loves me enough to expose me and heal me. Isn't that a great definition of love: to be known for who we really are and still to be loved in spite of all our sins! That kind of love continues to give joy to my heart and draws me to love him more and more.

It was an act of humility for me to make the decision to submit myself to prayer, but I knew that the enemy hated a humble spirit, and I knew God would not despise or reject such an attitude. Psalm 51:17 says, "The sacrifices of God are a broken spirit; a broken and contrite heart, O God, you will not despise." I was surely broken . . . right where God could help me: humble, helpless and hurting.

Even though the Lord had promised healing, I was beginning to understand that the healing would be a process, because I had some things the Lord wanted me to learn. Although the victory would be sure, the price would be faith and persistence. I had hoped for an instantaneous miracle, but that wasn't going to happen. Many examples of healing in the scriptures were of those who waited years for the appointed time of the Messiah, and yet they never lost hope. They never lost the expectation that Jesus could heal them and that their time would come. A common attitude they all shared was that each of them was desperate; their pleas for help were out of that place of desperation, and they knew where their help was from. God is always on time, and the sequence of events is in his hands. God allows us to go through seasons of desolation and humbling, so he can perfect our spiritual strength and develop character.

Additionally, there are no shortcuts to the development of strength and character. The Lord graciously allows challenges in our lives so that we increase our dependence upon him and we grow and develop spiritual muscle. I didn't like this training and discipline, but I needed a new perspective on the value of God's pruning and purging process. I could not allow myself to become a victim. Rather, I needed to become a mighty warrior and prepare for battle. This was a test and a tremendous opportunity to grow. I felt helpless, frail and frightened, far from being a victorious warrior. I began to understand the value of this time of trial, and as I could accept the situation I was more at peace and I even experienced times of feeling thankful. That was a miracle in itself! The weaker I got, the more opportunity for him to be strong in me, building the temple; a place for more of his presence. The words of 1 Peter 5:6–10 kept coming back to me:

> Humble yourselves, therefore, under God's mighty hand, that he may lift you up in due time . . . And the God of all grace, who called you to his eternal glory in Christ, after you have suffered a little while, will himself restore you and make you strong, firm and steadfast.

My idea of "a little while" and the Lord's idea were quite different. He did continually remind me of the value of this season of life because of the lessons I was learning. Again, this scripture came to life for me as the Lord began to reveal to me the spiritual implications of warfare that had both hindered me and would prove to be an asset as the healing progressed.

God is a God of restoration. I began to immerse myself in the scriptures and lay hold of the promises. The Bible truly became "life and medicine to my flesh." Although I would have preferred to work this out with the Lord alone, the act of humility was to continually submit myself to group prayer. I made an appointment for prayer with my pastor and elders, as directed in the Bible. I continued to take an inventory of my life from conception forward and began developing a list of circumstances in my life that were potential areas in need of healing: emotional, spiritual, mental and physical. Many family-of-origin issues continued to come to light. From that time on, I arranged to be in a prayer group or prayer counseling weekly, and to this day the practice of this discipline continues. The Lord intended for his church to be a safe haven and a refuge for those who have suffered the hardships and heartaches of life. Everyone wants to be loved and accepted and to know that there is mercy and forgiveness for all of our sins and failures.

What a calling for the church, that we would represent Jesus here on earth to the lost and hurting, moving and functioning in his love to offer signs, wonders and miracles to a dying world. In my past I have had some hurtful experiences in the church and the Lord wanted me to experience his healing among the faithful believers, in the midst of his servants where the liberty of the ministry of the Holy Spirit was free to move.

Such was the case and my experience with people of God who ministered to me through prayer. Today, I value more than ever the covenant relationship we have as believers and the commitment we have to one another. It is imperative that I have people around me who will love and care for me, pray for me and hold me accountable. I believe this is the plan God has for his church. His love, hands and mercy extended to each other, offering God's love and acceptance so that the world would know us by our love we have for each other. It is that agape, an unconditional love that is foreign to the world, and yet it is this love that will testify to the living God. The ability to share one's fears and problems leads to relief and healing. We all have our shortcomings, failures, and sins, but we will learn to love one another, encouraging one another, even more so as the days become darker, more sinful and challenging.

James 4:16–17 says, "Therefore confess your sins to each other and pray for each other so that you may be healed. The prayer of a righteous man is powerful and effective." The value of confession to another is that it breaks through the fears of rejection and hurt. Usually without confession to another there is no healing, because the wall of fear of being rejected is still there, blocking you from receiving love from God and others. God was calling me to a life characterized by the attitude of humility, which is an open, flowing and honest vulnerability before God and others. This was a challenge to all I had known and grown up with. God was at work, transforming my mindset and understanding.

**Personal reflection:**

Be willing to take a fearless, searching inventory of your life, both spiritual and moral. Bring these issues before the Lord. I make an effort to take inventory on a regular basis and develop a discipline of keeping short accounts with the Lord. Before bed at night I find I like to reflect over the day and seek the Lord as to any negative thoughts, attitudes or circumstances that need confession. Confession is good for the soul. 1 John 1:9–10: "If we claim to have fellowship with him yet walk in the darkness, we lie and do not live by the truth. But if we walk in the light, as he is in the light, we have fellowship with one another and the blood of Jesus, his Son, purifies us from all sin." Continue to take personal inventory of your life in the areas of the spirit, body and mind/emotions/soul.

1. What is your definition of humility? How does this aspect of character emanate from your life?

2. To what degree are you able to trust other believers in the body of Christ? List those friends with whom you have covenant relationship and could turn to in a time of need.

3. Compile a list of people you would like to ask to pray for you and minister to your spiritual needs.

4. As you pray and seek the Lord, ask the Holy Spirit to show you any areas of your life that have not been cleansed or healed by his presence. God began to bring up many areas of my life and show me where I needed his healing, forgiving presence. His purpose is not for condemnation but for freedom, strength, love, righteousness and joy. Take note of what he shows you.

## PERSONAL INVENTORY

| SPIRITUAL | EMOTIONAL | PHYSICAL |
|---|---|---|
| ex: unforgiveness toward God because of my father's death | ex: unresolved grief over father's death. Anger, fear, guilt, shame | ex: change my diet, identify all foods causing allergies |
|  |  |  |
|  |  |  |
|  |  |  |
|  |  |  |
|  |  |  |

Dear Lord,

You know me better than I know myself because you made me and you have seen all the experiences I have known to this time. Lord, I entrust myself to your care and believe that as I surrender all these areas of my life to you; you will begin the healing process. I am willing to face any dark, hidden faults in the inner most parts of my being known to you alone. Please shed the light of the Holy Spirit upon me and bring me to the place of wholeness, peace and restoration that you alone can accomplish. Thank you for your great mercy and love always offered so freely to me. Please give me the courage I need to walk through this process. Your loving daughter.

---

[1] Max Gerson, M.D., A Cancer Therapy: Results of Fifty Cases (Bonita, CA: The Gerson Institute, 1990), pg. 16.

[2] Linda Rector-Page, N.D., Ph.D., Healthy Healing (Sacramento, CA: Spilmen Printing Co., 1990), page 32.

[3] Anne Frahm, Cancer Battle Plan (Colorado Springs, CO: Ninon Press, 1992), pg. 102.

# Emotional Healing

**My Father's Heart**

The team continued to grow and now consisted of healthcare providers, a prayer ministry team and a cancer support group. As I continued to take inventory and as the Holy Spirit began to shed light upon my life, I could see how faithful God had been throughout the years, especially during some traumatic events in my life.

As I reflected over the past years of my life I was more aware of the fact that since I had come to have a personal relationship with Jesus, my entire perspective had changed. Suddenly, with the Holy Spirit at the helm, the whole world—including my personal world—took a dramatic paradigm shift and has not been the same since. Along with that shift came a change in behaviors, values and priorities. The scriptures say, "All things become new" (2 Corinthians 5:17). "Therefore, if anyone is in Christ, he is a new creation; the old has gone, the new has come!"

Certainly at the moment of salvation, God began a work in me that has continued. I had become adopted into the household of God; in essence I had a new family and especially a new Father. Learning to relate to my heavenly Father has been the key to my identity, my healing and my continued growth. Fortunately for me, I was able to receive the love of my heavenly father, which I could never remember having known from my earthly father.

Over time the Lord has caused our father-daughter relationship to develop and deepen. For those of us who have come from toxic or dysfunctional homes where the father was absent, abusive or negligent, accepting the love of the heavenly Father may present a challenge. Our natural response is to transfer our experience with our earthly fathers over to our heavenly Father. I believe the heart of God is that all of us come to him with the faith of a child and be able to receive his love as children, unadulterated by our life experience.

I shared the spiritual implications of the death of my father when I was nine years old. In addition to the spiritual issues I needed to address, there were emotional issues, as well. I learned unhealthy, false ways of dealing with emotions in my family. Losing a parent at a young age in a sudden, tragic event is a trauma representing a significant emotional loss. Not only was his death a loss, but the event itself was traumatic. The loss of my father left me with the feeling that I had been stripped of a protective covering I had always known. Now I was alone, feeling vulnerable. My sisters and I did not attend the funeral, and there was no further discussion about him. My mother, now alone and by herself with three little girls, handled the situation as well as she knew how, and that was to put this painful memory behind her and move on with life. Because of all the pain my mother carried, she never would talk about my father, and we never had the opportunity to grieve his death. My mother could not endure our pain, because it would tap into the grief she was carrying. I remember one time quite clearly, when my mother donated flowers to the church in honor of my father. When the pastor mentioned my father's name and talked briefly about him, my emotions came to the surface and I started to cry. My mother's way of handling the situation was to reprimand me for the tears. She reached over and grabbed my arm and pinched me until I stopped crying. I got the message that to grieve was wrong and unacceptable. Early on in life I determined that grief was not something to be felt or acknowledged, and certainly not to be displayed publicly. During those early childhood years growing up, I remember how difficult it was when a new child came to school. Of course everyone always wanted to know what my father did. I would avoid any new children, because I couldn't even mention my father had died without the pain and grief wanting to well up and seep out into the open. Over the years I got better at suppressing and stuffing that grief, and soon it was no longer like a raw wound throbbing with acute pain. In some ways it became a chronic situation that was never healed. What I didn't realize is that because that wound did not properly heal, it would resurface later, causing greater infection and toxicity.

Emotional healing was clearly a priority on God's agenda. He was determined to lift my burden of grief, heal the brokenhearted and teach me new, healthy ways of dealing with emotionally painful situations.

Maybe there is significance to the order of restoration starting with the spirit, then the soul and finally the body. Perhaps in that order we are made whole. At least that seemed to be the way God began the operation. At any rate, after coming to the Lord and receiving his Spirit, he began to remedy my emotions.

The Holy Spirit was able to break through the walls of protection I erected early on in life to protect myself from my own emotions. These walls kept me from intimacy and emotional honesty with others. First the Lord would draw me to an intimate relationship with himself and teach me what it would be like to have intimacy with others. My heavenly father began to reveal aspects of my life that needed addressing.

One of the first and most significant issues to be dealt with was the impact of growing up in an alcoholic home and all the unhealthy behaviors that accompany this family system. Just because I did not become an alcoholic, I had not escaped the impact of the disease. It is true that alcoholism is a family disease: everyone is affected by it. After exposing the grief of my father's death, I began to learn about the impact of the family into which I was born. Indeed, I was carrying a heavy burden of grief.

The dam was beginning to crack. Tears began to flow. I was reassured that the tears were healing. It was very uncomfortable for me to become vulnerable and release the pain, because it was in direct opposition to what I had been taught and had learned during the course of my life to this point. The work of uncovering all the grief and conflicts in my life became extremely important to my well-being. My heavenly father was going to draw me by his love and begin to reveal all the burdens my heart was carrying. By exposing and releasing all the conflict in my soul, my body would begin to use my life energy and direct it to overcoming the cancer. I learned that a lack of emotional outlet is a common theme in the histories of cancer patients. People who are forthright and honest with their emotions survive adversity better than those who are emotionally constricted. Unexpressed feelings suppress the immune system.

Dr. Caroline Bedell Thomas of John Hopkins University Medical School concluded that the personality traits of cancer patients were almost identical to those students who later committed suicide. "Almost all cancer patients throughout their lives had been restricted in expressing emotion, especially aggressive emotions related to their own needs."[1] God was beginning to transform my understanding of who I was in him, including the emotions he had built into my being.

**Journal entry:**

Dear Father,
You are indeed a most loving heavenly father, one with whom I am becoming more acquainted and familiar. Our relationship is entirely new, and even foreign to me and at times I am uncomfortable and guarded. If you will continue to show me how much you love me I know I will learn to trust you more and more. I appreciate your willingness to show me personally how you care for me and not just read about it in your word. Those little examples everyday how you talk to me and touch me through your presence is comforting and reassuring for me. I'm not sure what the future holds but you do and I am trusting you to bring me into a place of complete restoration and hope. Without you I cannot imagine experiencing all this upheaval and chaos. You alone can bring order and purpose to my life and because it is your nature you will do just that. You're my healer, my redeemer, my protector and my hope. You've promised that you would not with hold any good thing from those who love you. Your word is true and you cannot lie so with you there is hope.
Love,
Gretchen

## The Art of Hope

(author, unknown)

> The well-known maxim, "While there is life there is hope" has deeper meaning in reverse:
> "While there is hope there is life."
> Hope comes first, life follows. Hope gives power to life. Hope rouses life to continue, to expand, to grow, to reach out, to go on.
> Hope sees a light were there isn't any.
> Hope lights candles in millions of despairing hearts.
> Hope is the miracle medicine of the mind. It inspires the will to live.
> Hope is the physician's strongest ally.
> Hope is man's shield and buckler against defeat.
> "Hope," wrote Alexander Pope, "springs eternal in the human breast." And as long as it does man will triumph and move forward.
> Hope never sounds retreat.
> Hope keeps the banners flying.
> Hope revives ideals, renews dreams, revitalizes visions.

## Personal reflections:

1. What was your family of origin like? Describe its healthy and unhealthy aspects.

2. What kind of an impact does a father have in a home? What was your relationship with your father?

3. What behaviors have you learned, in order to provide protection for yourself?

4. How would you assess your level of intimacy with God and others? Do these levels coincide?

5. When you are feeling helpless and hopeless, where does your strength come from?

# Continue to Persevere

As I pursued my healing by gathering and trying to understand the collaborative research from around the world, I was amazed how God was continually dealing with me in the areas of my mind and emotions. I had always hoped God would instantaneously heal me, intervening in a supernatural way to correct my problem so I could get on with my life. Well, it became obvious to me that this was going to be the "getting on with my life" part. No doubt about it, God had many lessons to teach me. In turn, I hoped, others would be encouraged and helped, as well. If I had not learned these lessons, I would only continue to live a life that would be inconsistent with the life of the spirit and only cause more damage in the future. My prayer became this: "Lord, please help me to nurture a teachable spirit."

Spiritual warfare was on the lesson plan, and it was not something I really wanted to deal with. But I was forced out of denial, and my reticence was over. Most spiritual battles are won in our awareness and understanding of the work of the enemy. The battle in the spiritual realm is consistent and ongoing, because our lives are the target of an enemy of God and the enemy of our souls. The evil one is always looking for those whom he might destroy. Sometimes I think there are periods of rest or time off for good behavior, but that mindset is wrong. I was getting a spiritual revelation of the enemy's purpose and destructive power. For me, the greatest and most challenging battle was that of the battle in the mind. The enemy thrives on torment and terror, because once a thought is planted and then nurtured, thoughts become beliefs, which lead to action, which may prove crippling or ultimately disabling. Therefore, thoughts needed to be dealt with immediately and decisively.

Those initial days after having received the diagnosis were characterized by a mental battle between believing God's word or listening to the spirit of death harassing and tormenting me. The words of the physician who gave me the diagnosis kept coming back to haunt and oppress me: "You are terminal, and most people die within three years." When I allowed those thoughts to permeate my mind, I found I was stricken with terror, unable to function. I would sink into an abyss of depression and despair, waiting for the worst to happen. I had nowhere else to turn, so I cried out to God. I kept reminding myself of the scripture and the promise the Lord had impressed upon my heart. I kept choosing to believe that I would not die but would live. One minute I could believe what God had told me, and then the next moment I would have a thought that it wasn't true, it wasn't for me, and on and on. A foreboding sense of death is one of the most troubling and persistent experiences common to those facing terminal illness. My mind was in constant turmoil as I kept challenging the lies and replacing those thoughts with the promises in God's word. I knew I needed to build my faith, and the way to do that was to feed upon and immerse myself in those promises.

A friend of mine taped all the healing verses, so I could listen as well as read scripture. I found I needed to say the scriptures out loud over and over until they began to settle into my heart and soul. This was particularly helpful, since at night I often had difficulty sleeping because of the negative thought processes. As I listened to the taped promises, I could no longer entertain the negative, fear- provoking messages that wanted to taunt me. I was being forced to dismantle the fortresses of my own fears and thoughts.

According to 2 Corinthians 10:5, "We demolish arguments and every pretension that sets itself up against the knowledge of God, and we take captive every thought to make it obedient to Christ." The word of God became my weapon of truth to tear down all the false assumptions and expectation, fears, doubts and terror.

The promises would keep my mind stayed on the truth and kept my heart at peace.

In addition, I read testimonies of people God had healed, and my faith was encouraged and began to grow. I saturated my mind with truth. Ephesians 4:11–18 says:

> *Put on the full armor of God so that you can take your stand against the devil's schemes. For our struggle is not against flesh and blood, but against the rulers, against the authorities, against the powers of this dark world and against the spiritual forces of evil in the heavenly realms. Therefore put on the full armor of God, so that when the day of evil comes, you may be able to stand your ground, and after you have done everything, to stand. Stand firm then, with the belt of truth buckled around your waist, with the breastplate of righteousness in place, and with your feet fitted with the readiness that comes from the gospel of peace. In addition to all this, take up the shield of faith with which you can extinguish all the flaming arrows of the evil one. Take the helmet of salvation and the sword of the Spirit, which is the word of God. And pray in the Spirit on all occasions with all kinds of prayers and requests. With this in mind, be alert and always keep on praying for all the saints.*

So, there really is an enemy, but God has not left us defenseless. The word of God became my weapon and sure defense against these lies, doubts and fears. Every time I was assaulted with fear and doubt, I reached for the promises of God and took my stand. I told myself I must choose what I was going to believe. As I continued to resist the lies, I realized I was growing in my understanding of the word and the power it had to transform my thinking process. In doing so, I began to strengthen my resolve as I continued to cling to and speak out the truth.

During those cold and lonely nights so deep with anguish, the word of God would sustain me. I had come to a place where I was utterly helpless. The only way I knew to fight back was to hear and know what the word said. I started memorizing Psalm 91. The word of God began to soothe my soul as a cooling balm, and

I was comforted more and more as I ate of those promises. Gradually, I felt an inner strength begin to anchor and sustain me. As the winds of the storm would continue to come I felt more grounded and rooted. The Lord spoke to me through those words and reassured me of his presence with me.

As time went on, I became more steadfast and firm about the conviction that somehow, some way this would all work out for not only God's glory but for my best as well. I began to have a peace, even if intermittently, and it would grow stronger in time. My strength was in direct proportion to the capacity in which I could take hold of the word of God and let it become alive within me. As I accepted the promises as my own, applying them to my situation, I grew in faith and strength. The word is very powerful, living and active. Hope, inspired from the word, began to take root in the deep recesses of my inner being. That hope watered the belief that a sense of divine destiny would emerge from this abyss. I was no longer feeling like such a victim in this turbulent storm of my life. I was reassured that God alone holds the number of my days in his hands and to God belongs escape from death. Psalm 68:20 says, "Our God is a God who saves; from the Sovereign Lord comes escape from death." I realized that the Lord would bring me to my appointment with death. Even that thought became a comfort and joy to me. As God's grace is sufficient for our day-to-day needs, it is also sufficient for our hour of death. So, in the worst case scenario, I could even come to some peace and resolution about dying. As I continued to know my Lord and trust him, the unknown became less frightening to me. Even if I had misunderstood the Lord and I would die, the thought of death became less tormenting to me through all this. Oh, the mysteries of God . . . knowing him and loving him with all my heart, I discovered, was the solution to all that concerned me.

**Power of Praise**

I learned early on when I had first come to know the Lord that I would always choose to worship him, giving him praise, especially in the midst of circumstances where I did not feel thankful.

Nurturing a worshipful, joyful heart must not depend upon my emotions. It becomes a choice, because of who God is.

Scriptures have not left us without some examples of those who, in the middle of struggles and destitution, made the choice to worship. There is the example of Job who said, "Though he slay me, yet will I praise him" (Job 13:15).

The prophet Habakkuk could say,

> *Though the fig tree does not bud and there are no grapes on the vine, though the olive crop fails and the fields produce no food, though there are no sheep in the pen and no cattle in the stall, yet I will rejoice in the Lord. I will be joyful in God my Savior* (Habakkuk 3:17).

How contrary to all I felt! I chose to worship the Lord in spite of my circumstances. God is always worthy of my praise, he is still on the throne, exalted far above all this disaster, and I knew he would make a way for me.

My way of worship was to pick up the guitar and sing songs from the scriptures. I discovered as I did so, miraculously I was lifted above those despairing thoughts and attitudes, and my focus became fixed upon the Almighty, who was able to do more than I could ever ask or imagine. Now that was miraculous. As I made worship a lifestyle, I realized that my heart remained soft and tender before the Lord. I was able to cry before him, tell him how I felt and confess my unbelief and anger.

Worship actually became my weapon against the onslaught of anger, bitterness, resentment, unforgiveness, self-pity, depression and so on. These destructive thoughts could not penetrate my heart, as long as I stayed focused on the Lord and refused to resort to self-imposed walls as a means of protecting my heart. The Lord himself would become my defense. Didn't he promise that he would cause all things (yes, *all* things) to work for good for those who love God and are called according to his purpose? Romans 8:28 says, "And we know that in all things God works for the good of those who love him, who have been called according to his purpose." That is good news!

Job 23:10 says, "(God) knows the way that I take; when he has tested me I will come forth as gold." Times of testing will come in order that our faith will be tested, tried and proven genuine. There is always reason to praise God. Don't let circumstances rob you of the joy, peace and comfort that come to the heart of a worshipper. God promises to keep you in peace as your mind is kept upon him . . . his promises of goodness, love and mercy. Call upon him for help in your time of need.

**Journal entry:**

Oh Father, give me the eyes of faith and an illumination of your revelation with understanding so I will only be strengthened, purified and sanctified through this season. By your grace, cause my heart to extol and worship you knowing that ultimately your good purpose will be made known. I do not see the entire picture and I do not know what is ahead but I have confidence that you are a loving God and will do all that is according to your plans and purposes for my life. Please help me to understand how I can become victorious over the schemes of the enemy as I determine to believe your word and am filled with your wisdom and understanding. The battle is yours.
Love,
Gretchen

**Personal reflections:**
1. How well do you feel you understand spiritual warfare? What is your provision against the schemes of the enemy? How do you undertake the battle?

2. Identify times of spiritual warfare in your life. Share how, during one of these times you overcame the enemy of your soul.

3. In what ways has the memorization of scripture been a help or benefit for you?

4. Write a letter or song of worship to the Lord. Focus your understanding of him as the victor over all the battles that may be raging in your life.

# Job's Friends Come to Visit

*All changes, even the most longed for, have their melancholy; for what we leave behind us is a part of ourselves; we must die to one life before we can enter into another!* —Anatole France, writer

It was a Thursday morning, a day I generally meet with my prayer group, and I was struggling to get going. I was quite depressed that day, feeling hopeless and despairing. Tuesday of that week, two friends had come by to pray for me. This was shortly after the death of my stepfather; on top of that, I was needing a blood transfusion because my red blood counts were so low. Over the past two years I had become more and more dependent upon blood transfusions, which was not a good sign.

This was during the six-week program of the detoxification process to rid my body of the poisons that had accumulated. Since my stepfather had just died, I was feeling emotionally grieved and simply exhausted from the struggle. Sometimes the battle to stay alive seemed like it would consume me, and I didn't know if I would have the strength to go on.

When my friends came over that Tuesday, they asked if they could pray for me in light of everything that was happening. I had agreed to let them come, against my better judgment. When they came to the door, they saw that I had been crying and was depressed. At that point, out of their own fears and desperation, they started to tell me why I was sick and to take my personal inventory. I call it my Job visitation. Anything I had ever experienced or struggled with was up for scrutiny and judgment.

There is always a risk when we are in intimate relationships with one another, since our shortcomings and struggles might be turned upon us. My reaction to their inquisition was to put up a wall inside and sink into silence. I could feel myself shutting down my emotions and freezing. These were all my old, unhealthy ways of handling my emotions.

Finally, after I could not listen to any more critical, angry interrogation, I asked them to leave. Then I collapsed into tears, not only because of the grief of my stepfather's death and my physical body in a weakened state, but now I felt betrayed by some close friends. I knew they meant well, but now this was one more issue I had to wrestle with. My heart was hurting, and the sense of betrayal and misunderstanding only compounded the pain.

Fortunately, through all these years I only experienced this one time when prayer and ministry was more destructive than constructive. We need to learn to minister effectively and graciously. Confrontation, bringing about conviction not condemnation, must always be accomplished in a loving, merciful way with the intention of restoring not destroying.

I knew I needed to let go of the offense I had felt and not allow any unforgiveness to take root. I had read plenty of the book of Job, so I knew the solution for me to was forgive them and pray for them, which I did. From that time on, I have become very selective about who I have pray for me. I believe such a decision is good wisdom. Some people are not gifted with compassion and skill, and some simply have not experienced life's pain and suffering. These people are probably not the best folks for a prayer ministry.

I share this with you, because I want to contrast that experience with an experience of friends who are prayer warriors in the area of comfort and praying for the sick and wounded. People can learn to pray for the sick and minister effectively. For this, skills and sensitivity are needed.

## Job's Friends Come to Visit

It was now Thursday, and there was no way I even wanted to get out of bed, much less go to a prayer meeting—especially with the recent memory of my Job experience! When I feel despairing and hopeless, I start to want to isolate myself and wallow in self-pity. Knowing my pattern and inclination, I determined that I would get ready and make sure I got to my prayer group meeting, realizing that a pity party was not a place for me to linger.

It must have been obvious to my friends and prayer partners that morning when I arrived for prayer, because my dear friends immediately started to pray for me. My friend Mary is a massage therapist, counselor and pastor who has also done extensive work with trauma victims. She suggested I get on her massage table. Each of my friends gathered around me and laid hands on me: one at my head, one at my waist and one at my feet. No one said anything except to invite the Holy Spirit to come and minister to me.

After about five minutes, I felt very relaxed and peaceful. The best I'd felt in a long time! I almost got up and thanked them, when suddenly I could feel a swell of emotion coming from deep within my body; I began to cry uncontrollably. My body began to constrict, and I moved into a fetal position, drawing my knees upward toward my head. I was experiencing some very deep emotional pain that had been trapped in my body and was now free to be released. Mentally, I tried to control the situation and fight the emotional flood that was consuming me, but I could not stop the waves of emotion that poured out of me.

My friends continued to minister to me, praying softly and gently while my body was releasing this emotional pain. They cursed the root of cancer, and my body responded dramatically. I had no conscious realization of a particular event or situation in my life, but I knew that healing was taking place. I was being freed of some oppression and more grief and sorrow.

The presence of the Lord and the love expressed by my friends was the environment I needed, as the Lord began to expose these areas of emotional wounds. I felt loved and accepted, and as I cried and released the pain I could feel the comfort and love of the Lord expressed through the hands of my dear friends. They continued to pray and minister to me, and after that time we were in awe of what God had done. They anointed me with oil and prayed that the Holy Spirit would seal and protect the healing he had just accomplished.

After that time I felt a sense of peace, relaxation and energy. Although I was exhausted, it was a good sense of exhaustion where the body feels relieved to have a burden lifted. I believe my body had been holding this grief in for many years, and it had required a great deal of energy and vitality to manage the load. As the Lord healed this wound, the energy required to maintain that secret baggage was now available to enhance the physical function of my body as needed elsewhere.

The body was never intended to use its vitality to manage and store grief and sorrow. I could tell the tremendous amount of energy associated with the grief, because the deep sobbing was forceful and explosive. At long last my body was able to cast off the grief and be free from having to spend life energy suppressing it. The word of the Lord in Isaiah 61:1 says:

> *The spirit of the Sovereign Lord is upon me to preach good news to the poor. He has sent me to bind up the brokenhearted, to proclaim freedom for the captives and release for the prisoner, to proclaim the year of the Lord's favor and the day of vengeance of our God, to comfort all who mourn, and provide for those who grieve in Zion, to bestow on them a crown of beauty instead of ashes, the oil of gladness instead of mourning, and a garment of praise instead of a spirit of despair.*

These words became a living reality for me as the Lord healed my broken heart, freed me from the oppression of the emotional pain and granted me gladness and praise instead of despair. I no longer visit those deep, dark, lonely places of despondency, because they are no longer there and have not been since this healing episode. God is so awesome and wonderful. Nothing is too difficult for him. The healing process, working out my salvation one day at a time, continues on, by his grace and mercy.

**Personal reflections:**

The following is a letter from Lori, a dear friend. This letter has been a great, encouraging inspiration for me whenever I read it. I share it with you, because this dear friend has mastered the gift of speaking from the heart, finding godly words of tenderness from the heart of our Father in heaven. Whenever I am feeling without purpose and destiny, I take out this letter from my dear friend Lori and let it minister to my heart. Notice how she takes biblical principles and identifies the character of God at work in a person's life. Take time to let these words of hope minister to you. Then write a letter to someone who needs to hear some heavenly hope and inspiration today.

Dear Gretchen!

We just spent the afternoon together at a show that was far from successful in financial terms, although fruitful and beneficial from a friendship point of view.

During my drive home, you were on my mind . . . and I find it important to share with you some thoughts. Most importantly how much I admire your courage when you are dealing with so many uncertainties in your life and your willingness to always have God as your cornerstone. You are one of the few people I deeply admire and respect in my life. You always find a kind word or share wisdom that is beyond your years and experience. You find a place in your heart to help those who are searching and are always open to an opportunity to learn.

The young man who came to the booth today where I was concerned for you . . . your words were "he needed someone to talk with and you felt blessed by your conversation." Where does your thoughtful and kind way come from? Does God really work that deeply in our hearts to find the goodness in people at all times, no matter what the consequences? You are a living testimony of this.

And the purpose for my letter is to request you to keep your fight up, not to let Satan create weak opportunities for you that may be disguised as an easy and comfortable way. Gretchen, I firmly believe God has blessed you with the challenges you face today with your health, your family and finances for a sound reason . . . your personal testimony. Unfortunately, I did not have the good fortune of knowing you when you were married and money was no issue. I only remember the thoughts you have shared and believe you were a much different person then than you are today.
God knows what sacrifices you have made for him and continue to do today. He loves you, admires you and regards you as his dear child. Because of your faithfulness, he will bring forth incredible opportunities for you to minister for his benefit and ultimately yours!

I have found a friendship with you that only happens once in a lifetime. Thank you for always being a testimony to me, helping me to see the opportunities where God can continue to bless his children. Because of you, Gretchen, I believe I am becoming a better person. For this I am forever grateful for your tenderness and kindness.

You are my sister in Christ, we can do this together. We can be strong together and work towards your life's purpose of being a testimony of what your life was like prior to the opportunities our precious heavenly Father has so graciously provided to help build character, fortitude and perseverance in your soul. You always had them deep within . . . they are now ready for the world to see.

Gretchen, when times are tough or days are dark, please know I am always here for you . . . your cheerleader, cheering you on. If you want me to be with you when the treatments are hard, just to hold your hand, I am there. Please know you can count on me!

Life would not be the same without you! My life is forever changed because of you, your strength, your fortitude and ability to rise above adversity. Thank you for showing me by your action, words and deeds, how being a Christian can truly be a miracle in one's life.

I love You!
Lori

# Physical Healing

**How Could Things Get Worse?**

The old adage goes, "Sometimes things get worse before they get better." Well, during the first six months of the detoxification process, my cancer markers hit the highest levels they have ever been: 9860. Just so you have an idea about the levels, the normal range is around 1500. It made it very difficult to press forward and believe I was doing the right thing. I needed to trust that even though the circumstances looked bleak, they would turn around. The environmental doctor assured me that as toxins and impurities were exiting the body storage fat, tissue and bones, they were dumping into the bloodstream and would cause blood counts to jump around, becoming unstable for a while.

I had been warned that it could take up to two or more years to get the toxins—including mercury, solvents, pesticides and PCBs—completely out of my system. After one year of faithful and diligent adherence to the detoxification regimen, I suddenly felt an increased energy level my body had not known previously.

There is a product used in Japan in conjunction with chemotherapy, radiation and surgery to increase natural killer cell activity in the immune system. I had recently read about the efficacy of this product and decided to try it. My natural killer cell activity was very low, vacillating between 13 and 17. Normal range is between 60 and 100. Natural killer cells help kill cancer, and after three months on this immune modifier, my natural killer cell activity reached levels as high as 95, leveling off at about 65. In conjunction with immune modifiers, I had recently read about the use of thalidomide in cancer therapy—in particular multiple myeloma—and decided that the side effects were minimal when taken on short-term basis. This is the same drug that caused such horrible birth defects in the 1960s. There is an interesting story behind the use of this drug for treating multiple myeloma, and I find it very encouraging. It is a perfect example of how one individual with a vision and determination can affect the lives of others.

Beth Wolmer was a Manhattan lawyer whose husband Ira had been diagnosed with multiple myeloma in 1995 at the age of 35. Dr. Ira Wolmer was a cardiologist, had undergone three bone marrow transplants and had tried an experimental vaccine, but nothing worked. Mrs. Wolmer was the advocate every cancer patient needs. She was always looking for something new and would routinely call scientists in their labs to find out what they were working on.

One of those scientists told Mrs. Wolmer about Dr. Judah Folkman, a researcher at Harvard Medical School, who has theorized that cancer may be treated by retarding angiogenesis, the growth of blood vessels that feed tumors. One of the substances under study in Dr. Folkman's laboratory was thalidomide. Mrs. Wolmer called Dr. Folkman late one Saturday night in his laboratory and asked him if he thought thalidomide might work against multiple myeloma: "It was like a light bulb went on."

By fall of 1997 Mrs. Wolmer had received permission to test thalidomide in Ira Wolmer. Although he died in March 1998, other patients have benefited by Mrs. Wolmer's advocacy for her husband. That kind of persistence produced good fruitful results. I am grateful for your efforts Mrs. Wolmer; thank you.

My thinking was that perhaps I could halt the cancer with the combination of reducing the tumor bulk by taking the thalidomide—which acts to cut off the blood supply—and the increased immune activity of the immune modifiers. In two months of the combined therapy, my proteins dropped from the high of 9860 to 1980, which is the lowest they have been in all these years of recovery.

I remain very optimistic and encouraged, because my physical body is getting stronger all the time. I continue on the offensive, maintaining diligent action on all fronts: physically, spiritually and in the areas of my mind and emotions. The fruits of all the time, energy and resources is becoming evident. Regaining health is a costly venture, but what are the alternatives?

This entire process that I have been through continues to teach me about the challenges to my health, life and well-being. God wants me to enjoy a prosperous, joyful, peaceful life, and I agree with his purposes. I have learned to respond to stresses and crisis in life far differently than I did as a child.

Since I have made the decision to change and grow, I have left behind my family of origin, with all those destructive and damaging behavior patterns. My decision to change and embrace a different value system has caused me to be ostracized from my family of origin. Although I mourn the loss of my family and loved ones, I know today that the best I can do for them is to pray for and bless them, knowing God is faithful to hear my prayers for the salvation of my household. He alone is able to bring it to pass.

My responsibility is to guard my heart against unforgiveness, bitterness and anger caused by their alienation and hostility toward me. The principle applies to all relationships in my life. I have been challenged with residual feelings of vengeance. I have a very strong sense of justice, and to be mistreated by my family has caused a great feeling of injustice in my heart. I need to have the faith to let it go, trusting God to act justly for all involved. By guarding my heart I keep my heart free from inroads the enemy of my soul would like to re-establish.

During this time when my cancer markers reached their highest levels, when my family completely ostracized me, I realized that in my own strength I was utterly helpless and powerless. I actually remember one day when I broke into laughter at my situation, recognizing the enemy's bizarre tactics. He had pushed me too far this time and exposed himself, and all I could do was laugh at how ridiculous my circumstances had become. Faith had taken root in my heart, and I knew God was going to intervene! The forces of hell were doing all they could to bring fear, torment, unbelief and despair into my life, but God was bigger than all these challenges. All I could do was stand firm and nurture the seed of faith that God was beginning to water in my spirit. In spite of how I felt, I made the decision to press into God, believing he is faithful to his word and his promises to me.

It was during this time that I attended a seminar hosted by my church, which featured the teaching and ministry of Claudio Friedzon. Claudio is the pastor of the King of Kings Church in Buenos Aires, Argentina. In 1992 his hunger for God led him to a deep encounter with the Holy Spirit that revolutionized his life and ministry.

A fresh anointing overflowed the meetings at the King of Kings Church in a glorious way. Thousands of people from all over the world went there to be renewed. His ministry has been characterized by a powerful manifestation of the Holy Spirit through signs and wonders and Christ-centered preaching based upon the word of God. Whenever he preaches, the end results are conversions, testimonies of miracles and deep spiritual renewal in both pastors and lay people. In keeping with my hunger and desperation for God, I went to every meeting during this conference. God never disappoints a hungry heart. Over the years I have come to recognize the power and presence of the Almighty, and frankly, nothing else really is satisfying.

On the final evening of teaching and ministry, Claudio shared from the passage in 2 Kings 5:1–16. This is the passage of Naaman, commander of the Aramean army, through whom God had given victory to Aram. Naaman was a great man in the sight of his master and highly regarded, a valiant soldier. But he had leprosy, which was an incurable disease. Elisha's reputation as a healer reached Naaman through his wife's Israelite maidservant, who had a simple faith and concern for Naaman.

Naaman went to the man of God and at first was outraged by Elisha's instructions to wash seven times in the Jordan River. Having considered the alternatives, however, his obedience to Elisha's simple instructions produced healing. Faith and obedience took its course, and when Naaman came up out of that water on the seventh dip he was healed.

Claudio proceeded to say: "Many of you have been praying for healing for years, and you have been obedient and faithful. I want you to know that the Lord says tonight is the seventh dip . . . when you come up from that water you will be healed." When those words came forth, the Holy Spirit came upon me with such force I could not sit up straight. I was overcome by the spirit of God with deep groans, sobbing as the spirit of God shattered fear and unbelief deep into the resources of every cell in my being, penetrating my body, soul and spirit. Just as Naaman *knew*, when he came up from that seventh dip and was healed that there was no other God apart from the God of Israel, I felt like a transformed vessel, and I knew God was healing me. That word *know* in Hebrew is *yada*, which means to know by observing and reflecting, and to know by experiencing. There is an experiential side to the cognitive knowing, so that the knowing is a personal, intimate encounter with the living God. Naaman had known of God from reputation and believed. But now, after a personal encounter he had a new awareness, discernment and comprehension of God.

After my seventh dip I too had a new and distinguished acquaintance with the Holy One. What a privilege. Is anything too difficult for him? Through all these situations God is building up the most holy faith that he has deposited in this clay vessel. May his great name be praised. God, in his sweet mercy kept challenging my unbelieving heart, kept encouraging me and showing me how faithful and true he is to his word. He is causing me to go from faith to faith as I am being strengthened day by day, encounter by encounter.

Psalm 84:5–7 reads: "Blessed are those whose strength is in you, who have set their hearts in pilgrimage. As they pass through the Valley of Baca, they make it a place of springs; the autumn rains also cover it with pools. They go from strength to strength till each appears before God in Zion." Over all these years as I have traveled through the "Valley of Baca," meaning "valley of weeping," God is fashioning me into the person he wants me to become. Through all the times and waste places of deprivation, grief and sorrow, God has been there to provide the pools of refreshing living water through his presence.

Setting my heart upon God, seeking him at all costs causes a change within me. A point of desperation can prove to be of great value. These encounters cause a reordering of priorities and bring about the sanctifying experience, which results in a cleansing and washing of my spirit. All the inner corruption, wrong thinking and defiling residue becomes exposed in his presence.

The cry of the psalmist becomes the cry of the suffering soul when he says, "It was good for me to be afflicted, so that I might learn your decrees." There is no way I would ever have had to face the innermost sanctuary of my heart if it had not been for the fiery furnaces of affliction, which has served to expose all these areas of my soul.

In the process of exposure I have learned the consequences of sinful thoughts and behaviors that have worked together to cause death in my soul. God is most concerned about the issues of the heart and the sins that bring alienation and separation from him. He never gives up on me. I am so grateful for his persistent love and pursuit of me. My heart rejoices at his goodness to me. As Paul says in 1 Thessalonians 5:23–24, "May God himself, the God of peace, sanctify you through and through. May your whole spirit, soul and body be kept blameless at the coming of our Lord Jesus Christ. The one who calls you is faithful, and he will do it."

# Peace at Last

*A heart at peace gives life to the body.*
—Proverbs 14:30

Fall is one of my most favorite times of the year; the season is changing from the fruitful harvest time of summer and moving into the rest of winter. There is a crisp chill in the air as the leaves and colors begin to change. Biblically, and in keeping with the Lord's schedule and timetable, this is the season of the High Holy days, a time of reflection and repentance. I like this season because to me represents newness and fresh beginnings. It is a time I focus on the Person, the plan and the character of the Holy One of Israel, recognizing his complete sovereignty over all of time, history and the details of my individual life. The feast of Trumpets teaches repentance, the Day of Atonement, redemption and Tabernacles, rejoicing. So all these thoughts were in the forefront of my mind as I meditated on Psalm 51 one day:

*Have mercy on me, O God, according to your unfailing love; according to your great compassion, blot out my transgressions. Wash away all my iniquity and cleanse me from my sin. For I know my transgressions, and my sin is always before me. Against you, you only, have I sinned and done what is evil in your sight, so that you are proved right when you speak and justified when you judge. Surely I have been a sinner from birth, sinful from the time my mother conceived me. Surely you desire truth in the inner parts. You teach me wisdom in the inmost place. Cleanse me with hyssop and I will be clean; wash me, and I will, be whiter than snow. Let me hear joy and gladness; let the bones you have crushed rejoice . . . Create in me a pure heart O God, and renew a steadfast spirit within me.*

This psalm has always been one of my favorite passages in scripture. Since I am passionate for truth, these words become my prayer, especially now in this season of reflection.

How, I wonder, can sin be so pervasive that even at conception and from birth we are sinners? Lord, how would I ever know what all my sinful thoughts, judgments and vows have been when I was yet an infant or small child? I certainly have no capacity to know what is in my heart. But you, by your Spirit, are able to search my heart and cleanse me from all unrighteousness. You have brought me through so much these past years, and I am at a place where physically I am better than I have been in quite some time. Perhaps it will be this year, a new season of life to complete the good work you have begun in my healing process. Once again, Lord, I humble myself before you and ask that your will be done.

During this time of year my prayer partner Mary and I had signed up to take a continuing education course in cranialsacral therapy. I have been particularly fascinated by the complexity of the human body, as well as the relationship between the body, soul and spirit as God has designed.

As I have journeyed these years through the process of my own healing, I have better understood the direct relationship between the parts of our being and how they all interconnect and relate to one another, for instance, the mind/emotional influence upon the physical health of the body. Science has yet to scientifically define such variables, but the reality exists. Likewise, the spiritual influence of good or evil has a profound influence upon our physical and mental wellness. The techniques of cranialsacral therapy enable the body to begin to release and identify memory of past trauma and abuse. I'm not sure how and why it happens, but time and again I have seen the power of the therapy to tap into body memory and subsequently see a person freed from the energy and power of negative assaults upon an individual.

It was during this course that I became aware that there was some more emotional healing in my heart that God was beginning to bring to light. Fortunately for me, my prayer partner, dear friend and colleague is also a therapist and pastor who is very gifted in ministry to the brokenhearted and people who have experienced trauma. We both agreed that at our next prayer meeting on Thursday, we would have the prayer group pray over me and see what God was doing

Of course, when we met for our next prayer group, there were three new women. I was uncomfortable with the new women, because I was feeling vulnerable about the possibility of becoming emotional during the ministry time. I made the decision that it was more important to be free than to worry about what strangers may think, so I agreed to get on the altar and ask for the cleansing work of the fire of God. My friend Mary led in the prayer and ministry time, directing the laying on of hands and explaining what was happening as they prayed and the Holy Spirit ministered.

By now I am beginning to recognize when I am getting in touch with deep, repressed emotional pain. I start to tremble and way down deep in my body, in the area of my bowels there begins to be a feeling like water breaking through a dam. It feels like a welling up and a bursting forth of emotion. Mary said these words to me: "Gretchen, the Lord has put before you life and death: choose life." When she said "Choose life," something inside of me rose up in powerful defiance and said "No!"

Time and again, that childlike voice within refused to accept life. Mary discerned that at some point in my development in the womb I had made a vow not to be born. By doing so, I had made a decision not to choose life and had carried that message in the form of a vow for my entire life to this point in time. How, I wondered, could such a decision, with such conviction, not affect every part of my being? While my grown-up, regenerated, Christ-centered part of me wanted the abundant life, there was a part of my heart that was un-regenerated and was choosing death. I was under the veil of a sinful vow I had made in the womb.

Mary has worked with many clients who have been freed from trauma and sin clear back to the moment of conception. It seems so unfair that an infant in the womb could be subject to sinful, evil assault, but the reality is that it does happen. I know that my father was a raging, belligerent alcoholic when he and my mother married. My mother alluded to the fact that he had been physically abusive and had committed adultery. I remember always feeling fearful and wanting to disappear and hide whenever I was around my father's family, because they all drank and the atmosphere was hostile and loud. When the enemy of our souls has the capacity to thwart the protective role of parents and bind them, then he has free access to the seed of the parents.

God made parents the protective agents in the lives of children. In his book *Ancient Paths*, Craig Hill notes:

> God gave protective measures in the Law of Moses. For the ancient people, he wanted to ensure that children would be blessed right from the time of conception.
>
> Identity of a child is blessed at the time of conception when two primary requirements are met:
> 1. The conception occurs between two people who have chosen to place themselves under God's protective authority through marriage, and
> 2. The child is wanted, accepted, and received.
>
> A child's identity can be cursed at the time of conception when the child is:
> 1. Conceived outside of wedlock, or
> 2. Not wanted, accepted and received, or considered an intrusion into the life of the mother.[1]

It all began to make sense to me, and I could believe that as an infant in the womb I decided that I did not want to be born, having sensed the great turmoil that would be awaiting me. Satan's intention is to distort or entirely replace the person God has called each of us to be. Any opportunity to rob, steal or destroy will be fully undertaken by our enemy.

As my friends were ministering to me and Mary was saying that I needed to choose life, I renounced the vow and received forgiveness. I could feel a release in my body and simultaneously deep from within me a spirit came up and out my mouth. Once again, having experienced a greater liberty, I felt washed, free from oppression and sensing new life within.

God is so good to me, continuing to cleanse me from all unrighteousness. Mary looked at me and I agreed, having had the same thought, that this was the root of the cancer in my body. I have always known that the Lord was leading me to pursue health and wholeness by getting to and identifying the root causes of my illness. I believe with all my heart that is the only way to treat disease, regardless of the physical symptoms. For me the journey has been complete and all encompassing in my body, soul and spirit.

I am convinced that in order to be healthy, functioning whole people, the sanctification process is an ongoing course of action throughout our lives. The body, soul and spirit is always subject to the assault of evil. By God's grace we have his Spirit at work within us to cleanse us from all ungodliness and unrighteousness on an ongoing basis. Just as the psalmist said, God desires truth "in the inward parts" . . . and he will bring truth to our inward parts if we humble ourselves and allow him to sanctify us.

Oh how great a love, what a God of wonder and might that he would reach across the darkness and night to draw my soul into his marvelous light . . . (Selah—meditate on this thought!) My love only grows more and more for my gracious, loving Savior.

I started my testimony by stating that even when destruction has taken a toll, the grace and mercy of God is able to bring restoration, healing and joy. In fact, this is what the Lord has done for me. God is willing to do good to all who seek him and call upon his name. In the last three chapters of Daniel, regarding the vision of the end times, the angel tells Daniel:

> *And some who are the most gifted in the things of God will stumble in those days and fall, but this will only refine and*

*cleanse them and make them pure until the final end of all their trials, at God's appointed time* (Dan. 11:35 TLB).

We also know from scripture that before Christ returns he will return for a church that has been purified, refined, spotless and pure.

Could it be that we are truly in those days when the grace of God is preparing his bride for his return? When we stumble or fall, perhaps it is a blessing and an opportunity for God to be manifest in our lives in greater measure. As we offer the circumstances up to him and allow him to consume us with his refining fires, God can burn out all the dross, sin and residue of this world.

Rejoice, rejoice, because the kingdom of God is at hand, and those who know their God will display strength and do mighty exploits. This is not a time to be passive but to take up your sword, which is the word of God, and contend for the blessings that have been promised for the people of the covenant. The battle can be fierce but Jesus has won the war. Our job is to press through until we realize the complete victory.

Every day is an opportunity to offer ourselves as those living sacrifices unto the Lord, allowing him to sanctify us and conform us more to his image. We are in a battle, but we have the victory. It does require that we continue to contend for that victory, but Christ Jesus our Lord has given us everything we need to be overcomers. We have overcome the enemy by the blood of the Lamb, the word of our testimony, and we have not loved our lives even unto death.

One day we will no longer contend for blessings, but we will live and abide in the kingdom of God when it is established here on earth in all of its fullness, with complete righteousness and justice, with our dear Lord as King of Kings and Lord of Lords. What a day that will be. Until then, be of good cheer, take heart and keep on contending . . . the promises and blessings belong to every child of God.

Today, I have, for the first time in more than eight and a half years (seems like a lifetime), and about one month after this last deliverance and healing, now reached a place of remission in my battle with multiple myeloma. It has been an extensive, difficult and severely trying time in my life. Never, never give up or lose heart. When I couldn't go on and believe, I always had someone who would stand in the gap for me with their faith and believe for me, encourage me and instill hope into my heart. I remain diligent and continue to be watchful on this front because cancer is such an insidious enemy.

Perseverance is just one of the valuable lessons I have learned. I continue to treasure and apply so many of the lessons I have gained, not turning back but continuing forward, onward and upward desiring to know God more all the time. I can wholeheartedly say that I am grateful for the experience of the last several years as God has brought me through the most severe testing and trial of my life. There are skills and knowledge I could never have acquired apart from the experience of on the job training. Most importantly, today I know my Lord, the lover of my soul in an intimate, tender way that means more to me than anything this world has to offer. He is everything to me. What is it that pleases him? Faith pleases him. It brings joy to my heart that my faith has grown these past eight years, and what better way to give back to him all that he has done for me? By blessing him I am blessed. This is a principle of the kingdom of God. May it come soon in all of its fullness.

I pray that you too may come to know him, his gracious tender loving mercy. God is good in all things and at all times. Bless his name.

---

[1] Craig Hill, The Ancient Paths (Family Foundations Publishing, 1992), pg. 59–60.

# Appendix

**Healing Prayer According to God's Word**

Begin to memorize the word of God. Take it in and let it bring life, truth and healing to your body, soul and spirit. I put the following affirmation and scriptures on tape and listened to them constantly until they became settled in my heart and mind.

"The word of God," according to John Hagee, "is the basis of every healing and every miracle in your life. Psalm 107:20 says: 'He sent forth his word and healed them.' The Bible says, 'Have faith in God; nothing is impossible for those who believe.' Faith comes by hearing and hearing by the word of God. Hear this confession and learn to speak it. In speaking the word of God, you release the electrifying power that raised Jesus from the grave."

Hagee continues with a prayer:

> Father, in the name of Jesus I confess your word concerning healing. As I do this I believe and say that your word will not return void, but it will accomplish what it says it will. Therefore I believe in the name of Jesus that I am being healed as I hear the word of God. It is written in your word that Jesus himself took our infirmities and bore our sicknesses; therefore with great boldness and confidence I say on the authority of the written word of God that I am redeemed from the curse of sickness, and I refuse to tolerate its symptoms. Satan, I speak to you in the name of Jesus that your principalities and powers, your spirits you have in present darkness and spiritual wickedness in heavenly places are bound from operating against me in anyway. I am the property of the

Lord Jesus Christ, I am a child of God and I give you no place in me. I dwell in the secret place of the Most High God. I abide, I remain stable and fixed under the shadow of the Almighty and his power is in me and no foe can withstand me. Now Father, because I reverence and fear you, I have the assurance that the angel of the Lord encamps about me and delivers me from every evil work. No evil will befall me, no plague or calamity shall come near my dwelling. I confess the word of God abides in me and delivers me perfect soundness of mind and wholeness in body and spirit from the deepest parts of my nature from my immortal spirit even to the joints and marrow of my bones. That word of God is medication and life to my flesh. For the law of the spirit of life operates in me and makes me free from the law of sin and death. I have on the whole armor of God and the shield of faith protects me from all the fiery darts of the wicked one. Jesus is my high priest and he is hearing my confession. I hold fast to this confession of faith through the word of God. I stand immovable and fixed in full assurance that I have health and healing in the name of the Lord Jesus Christ. My healing has been purchased through the blood of Christ and as I hear these healing scriptures the anointing power of the Lord is being released into my life. It is attacking my disease and I am being healed.

Meditate on these scriptures about healing:

**Luke 17:12–14** As he was going into a village, ten men who had leprosy met him. They stood at a distance and called out in a loud voice, "Jesus, Master, have pity on us!" When he saw them, he said, "Go, show yourselves to the priests." And as they went they were cleansed.

**Acts 3:2–8** Now a man crippled from birth was being carried to the temple gate called Beautiful, where he was put every day to beg from those going into the temple courts. When he saw Peter and John about to enter, he asked them for money. Peter looked straight at him as did John. Then Peter said, "Look at us!" So the man gave them his attention, expecting to get something from them.

Then Peter said, "Silver or gold I do not have, but what I have I give you. In the name of Jesus Christ of Nazareth, walk." Taking him by the right hand, he helped him up, and instantly the man's feet and ankles became strong. He jumped to his feet and began to walk. Then he went with them into the temple courts, walking and jumping, and praising God.

**Acts 10:34–35** I now realize how true it is that God does not show favoritism but accepts men from every nation who fear him and do what is right.

**Matt 20:30–34** Two blind men were sitting by the roadside, and when they heard that Jesus was going by, they shouted, "Lord, Son of David, have mercy on us!" Jesus stopped and called them. "What do you want me to do for you?" He asked. "Lord," they answered, "we want our sight." Jesus had compassion on them and touched their eyes. Immediately they received their sight and followed him.

**Acts 14:8–10** In Lystra there sat a man crippled in his feet, who was lame from birth and had never walked. He listened to Paul as he was speaking. Paul looked directly at him, saw that he had faith to be healed and called out, "Stand up on your feet!" At that, the man jumped up and began to walk.

**Matt 8:14–16** When Jesus came into Peter's house, he saw Peter's mother-in-law lying in bed with a fever. He touched her hand and the fever left her, and she got up and began to wait on him. When evening came, many who were demon-possessed were brought to him, and he drove out the spirits with a word and healed all the sick.

**Matt 8:5–10,13** When Jesus had entered Capernaum, a centurion came to him, asking for help. "Lord," he said, "my servant lies at home paralyzed and in terrible suffering." Jesus said to him, "I will go and heal him." The centurion replied, "Lord, I do not deserve to have you come under my roof. But just say the word and my servant will be healed. For I myself am a man under authority with soldiers under me. I tell this one, 'go.' And he goes, and that one 'Come,' and he comes. I say to my servant, 'Do this,' and he does it." When Jesus heard this, he was astonished and said to those following him, "I tell you the truth. I have not found anyone in Israel with such great faith." Then Jesus said to the centurion, "Go! It will be done just as you believed it would."

**Proverbs 3:5–8** Trust in the Lord with all your heart and lean not on your own understanding; in all your ways acknowledge him, and he will make your paths straight. Do not be wise in your own eyes; fear the Lord and shun evil. This will bring health to your body and nourishment to your bones.

**Isaiah 53:5** But he was pierced for our transgressions, he was crushed for our iniquities; the punishment that brought us peace was upon him, and by his wounds we are healed.

**Matt 14:35–36** And when the men of that place recognized Jesus, they sent word to all the surrounding country. People brought all their sick to him and begged him to let the sick just touch the edge of his cloak and all who touched him were healed.

**Psalm 103:1–3** Praise the Lord, O my soul; all my inmost being, praise his holy name. Praise the Lord, O my soul, and forget not all his benefits. He forgives all my sins and heals all my diseases; he redeems my life from the pit and crowns me with love and compassion.

**Matt 4:23–24** Jesus went throughout Galilee, teaching in their synagogues, preaching the good news of the kingdom, and healing every disease and sickness among the people. News about him spread all over Syria, and people brought to him all who were ill with various diseases, those suffering severe pain. The demon-possessed, the epileptics and the paralytics, and he healed them.

**Matt 8:2–3** A man with leprosy came and knelt before him and said, "Lord, if you are willing, you can make me clean." Jesus reached out his hand and touched him. "I am willing", he said. "Be clean!"

**Romans 8:11** And if the Spirit of him who raised Jesus from the dead is living in you, he who raised Christ from the dead will also give life to your mortal bodies through his Spirit, who lives in you.

**John 5:2–9** Now there is in Jerusalem near the Sheep Gate a pool, which in Aramaic is called Bethesda and which is surrounded by five covered colonnades. Here a great number of disabled people used to lie-the blind, the lame the paralyzed. One who was there had been an invalid for thirty-eight years. When Jesus saw him lying there and learned that he had been in this condition for a long time, he asked him, "Do you want to get well?" "Sir," the invalid replied, "I have no one to help me into the pool when the water is stirred. While I am trying to get in someone else goes down ahead of me." Then Jesus said to him, "Get up! Pick up your mat and walk." At once the man was cured; he picked up his mat and walked.

**Luke 13:10–13** On a Sabbath Jesus was teaching in one of the synagogues, and a woman was there who had been crippled by a spirit for eighteen years. She was bent over and could not straighten up at all. When Jesus saw her, he called her forward and said to her, "Woman, you are set free from your infirmity." Then he put his hands on her, and immediately she straightened up and praised God.

**Luke 4:18–19** The Spirit of the Lord is on me, because he has anointed me to preach good news to the poor, he has sent me to proclaim freedom for the prisoners and recovery of sight for the blind, to release the oppressed, to proclaim the year of the Lord's favor."

**Isaiah 58:6–9** Is not this the kind of fasting I have chosen: to loose the chains of injustice and untie the cords of the yoke, to set the oppressed free and break every yoke? Is it not to share your food with the hungry and to provide the poor wanderer with shelter-when you see the naked, to clothe him and not to turn away from your own flesh and blood? Then your light will break forth like the dawn, and your healing will quickly appear; then your righteousness will go before you, and the glory of the Lord will be your rear guard. Then you will call and the Lord will answer; you will cry for help and he will say: Here am I. If you do away with the yoke of oppression with the pointing finger and malicious talk, and if you spend yourselves in behalf of the hungry and satisfy the needs of the oppressed, then your light will rise in the darkness, and your night will become like the noonday.

**3 John 1–2** Dear friend, I pray that you may enjoy good health and that all may go well with you, even as your soul is getting along well.

**Matt 9:27–30** As Jesus went on from there, two blind men followed him, calling out, "Have mercy on us, Son of David!" When he had gone indoors, the blind men came to him, and he asked them, "Do you believe that I am able to do this?" "yes, Lord," they replied. Then he touched their eyes and said, "According to your faith will it be done to you" and their sight was restored

**Proverbs 4:20–27** My son, pay attention to what I say; listen closely to my words. Do not let them out of your sight, keep them within your heart; for they are life to those who find them and health to a man's whole body. Above all else, guard your heart, for it is the wellspring of life. Put away perversity from your mouth; keep corrupt talk far from your lips. Let your eyes look straight ahead, fix your gaze directly before you. Make level paths for your feet and take only ways that are firm. Do not swerve to the right or the left; keep your foot from evil.

**Luke 8:41–55** Just then a man named Jairus, a ruler of the synagogue, came and fell at Jesus' feet pleading with him to come to his house because his only daughter, a girl of about twelve, was dying. As Jesus was on his way, the crowds almost crushed him. And a woman was there who had been subject to bleeding for twelve years, but no one could heal her. She came up behind him and touched the edge of his cloak, and immediately her bleeding stopped. "Who touched me?" Jesus asked. When they all denied it, Peter said, "Master, the people are crowding and pressing against you." But Jesus said, "Someone touched me; I know that power has gone out from me." Then the woman, seeing that she could not go unnoticed, came trembling and fell at his feet. In the presence of all the people, she told why she had touched him and how she had been instantly healed. Then he said to her, "Daughter, your faith has healed you. Go in peace." While Jesus was still speaking someone came from the house of Jairus, the synagogue ruler. "Your daughter is dead," he said. "Don't bother the teacher any more." Hearing this, Jesus said to Jairus, "Don't be afraid; just believe, and she will be healed." When he arrived at the house of Jairus, he did not let anyone go in with him except Peter, John and James, and the child's father and mother. Meanwhile, all the people were wailing and mourning for her. "Stop wailing," Jesus said. "She is not dead but asleep." They laughed at him, knowing that she was dead. But he took her by the hand and said, "My child, get up!" Her spirit returned, and at once she stood up. Then Jesus told them to give her something to eat. Her parents were astonished, but he ordered them not to tell anyone what had happened.

**Mark 16:17–18** And these signs will accompany those who believe: In my name they will drive out demons; they will speak in new tongues; they will pick up snakes with their hands; and when they drink deadly poison, it will not hurt them at all; they will place their hands on sick people, and they will get well.

**James 5:14–15** Is any one of you sick? He should call the elders of the church to pray over him and anoint him with oil in the name of the Lord. And the prayer offered in faith will make the sick person well; the Lord will raise him up. If he has sinned he will be forgiven.

**Deuteronomy 7:15** The Lord will keep you free from every disease. He will not inflict on you the horrible diseases you knew in Egypt but will inflict them on all who hate you.

**1 Peter 2:24** He himself bore our sins in his body on the tree, so that we might die to sins and live for righteousness; by his wounds you have been healed.

**Exodus 15:26** "If you listen carefully to the voice of the Lord your God and do what is right in his eyes, if you pay attention to his commands and keep all his decrees, I will not bring on you any of the diseases I brought on the Egyptians, for I am the Lord who heals you."

**Luke 4:40** When the sun was setting the people brought to Jesus all who had various kinds of sickness, and laying his hands on each one, he healed them.

**Acts 10:38** . . . how God anointed Jesus of Nazareth with the Holy Spirit and power, and how he went around doing good and healing all who were under the power of the devil, because God was with him.

**Luke 6:19** and the people all tried to touch him, because power was coming from him and healing them all.

**Psalm 107:20** He sent forth his word and healed them; he rescued them from the grave.

**Psalm 30:2** O Lord my God, I called to you for help and you healed me.

**Matthew 8:17** This was to fulfill what was spoken through the prophet Isaiah: "he took up our infirmities and carried our diseases."

**Jeremiah 33:6** Nevertheless, I will bring health and healing to it; I will heal my people and will let them enjoy abundant peace and security.

**Psalm 18:30** As for God, his way is perfect; the word of the Lord is flawless, he is a shield for all who take refuge in him.

**Psalm 23:3** He restores my soul. He guides me in paths of righteousness for his name's sake.

**Psalm 25:3** No one whose hope is in you will ever be put to shame, but they will be put to shame those who are treacherous without excuse.

**Psalm 34:17** The righteous cry out, and the Lord hears them; he delivers them from all their troubles.

**Psalm 55:22** Cast your cares on the Lord and he will sustain you; he will never let the righteous fall.

**Psalm 57:1** Have mercy on me, O God, have mercy on me, for in you my soul takes refuge. I will take refuge in the shadow of your wings until the disaster has passed.

**Psalm 86:1** Hear, O Lord, and answer me, for I am poor and needy.

**Psalm 91:5–8** You will not fear the terror of night, nor the arrow that flies by day, nor the pestilence that stalks in darkness, nor the plague that destroys at midday. A thousand may fall at your side, ten thousand at your right hand but it will not come near you. You will only observe with your eyes and see the punishment of the wicked.

**Psalm 112:7** He will have no fear of bad new; his heart is steadfast, trusting in the Lord.

**Psalm 116:8–9** For you, O Lord have delivered my soul from death, my eyes from tears, my feet from stumbling, that I may walk before the Lord in the land of the living.

**Psalm 119:50** My comfort in my suffering is this: Your promise renews my life.

**Psalm 119:16** I delight in your decrees; I will not neglect your word.

**Romans 8:13** I consider that our present sufferings are not worth comparing with the glory that will be revealed in us.

**Matthew 21:22** If you believe, you will receive whatever you ask for in prayer.

**1 John 4:4** You, dear children, are from God and have overcome them because the one who is in you is greater than the one who is in the world.

**Romans 10:17** Consequently, faith comes from hearing the message, and the message is heard through the word of Christ.

**Hebrews 11:1** Now faith is being sure of what we hope for and certain of what we do not see.

**Mark 9:23** "If you can?" said Jesus. "Everything is possible for him who believes."

**Psalm 118:8** It is better to take refuge in the Lord than to trust in man.

**Matthew 13:58** And he did not do many miracles there because of their lack of faith.

**Psalm 91:9–11** If you make the Most High your dwelling—even the Lord, who is my refuge—then no harm will befall you, no disaster will come near your tent. For he will command his angels concerning you to guard you in all your ways

**Psalm 118:17** I will not die but live and will proclaim what the Lord has done.

**Psalm 91:14–16** "Because he loves me," says the Lord, "I will rescue him; I will protect him, for he acknowledges my name. He will call upon me and I will answer him; I will deliver him and honor him. With long life will I satisfy him and show him my salvation."

**Psalm 107:20** He sent forth his word and healed them; he rescued them from the grave

**Luke 1:38** "I am the Lord's servant," Mary answered. "May it be done to me as you have said."

**Acts 10:34** Then Peter began to speak: "I now realize how true it is that God does not show favoritism but accepts men from every nation who fear him and do what is right."

**Ephesians 3:20** Now to him who is able to do immeasurably more than all we ask or imagine, according to his power that is at work within us, to him be glory in the church and in Christ Jesus throughout all generations, for ever and ever! Amen.

**John 10:10** The thief comes only to steal and kill and destroy; I have come that they may have life, and have it to the full.

**Luke 10:9–13** Heal the sick who are there and tell them, "The kingdom of God is near you." But when you enter a town and are not welcomed, go into its streets and say, "Even the dust of your town that sticks to our feet we wipe off against you. Yet be sure of this: The kingdom of God is near. I tell you, it will be more bearable on that day for Sodom than for that town. Woe to you, Chorazin! Woe to you, Bethsaida! For if the miracles that were performed in you had been performed in Tyre and Sidon, they would have repented long ago, sitting in sackcloth and ashes. But it will be more bearable for Tyre and Sidon at the judgment than for you."

**Mark 11:22–24** "Have faith in God" Jesus answered. "I tell you the truth, if anyone says to this mountain, 'Go, throw yourself into the sea' and does not doubt in his heart and believes that what he says will happen, it will be done for him. Therefore I tell you, whatever you ask for in prayer, believe that you have received it, and it will be yours".

**Mark 10:27** Jesus looked at them and said, "With man this is impossible, but not with God; all things are possible with God."

**Proverbs 7:1–3** My son, keep my words and store up my commands within you. Keep my commands and you will live; guard my teaching as the apple of your eye. Bind them on your fingers; write them on the tablet of your heart.

**Romans 12:11–12** Never be lacking in zeal, but keep your spiritual fervor, serving the Lord. Be joyful in hope, patient in affliction, faithful in prayer.

**Jeremiah 29:11–14** "For I know the plans I have for you," declares the Lord, "plans to prosper you and not to harm you, plans to give you hope and a future. Then you will call upon me and come and pray to me, and I will listen to you. You will seek me and find me when you seek me with all your heart. I will be found by you," declares the Lord, "and will bring you back from captivity. I will gather you from all the nations and places where I have banished you," declares the Lord, "and will bring you back to the place from which I carried you into exile."

**Isaiah 57:18** I have seen his ways, but I will heal him; I will guide him and restore comfort to him.

**Isaiah 54:13–17** All your sons will be taught by the Lord, and great will be your children's peace. In righteousness you will be established. Tyranny will be far from you; you will have nothing to fear, terror will be far removed; it will not come near you. If anyone does attack you it will not be my doing; whoever attacks you will surrender to you. See, it is I who created the blacksmith who fans the coals into flame and forges a weapon fit for its work. And it is I who have created the destroyer to work havoc; no weapon forged against you will prevail, and you will refute every tongue that accused you. This is the heritage of the servants of the Lord, and this is their vindication from me declares the Lord.

**Isaiah 45:22** Turn to me and be saved, all you ends of the earth; for I am God, and there is no other.

**Proverbs 4:10** Listen, my son, accept what I say, and the years of your life will be many.

**Psalm 145:13** Your kingdom is an everlasting kingdom, and your dominion endures through all generations. The Lord is faithful to all his promises and loving toward all he has made.

**1 John 1:5–8** This is the message we have heard from him and declare to you; God is light; in him there is no darkness at all. If we claim to have fellowship with him yet walk in the darkness, we lie and do not live by the truth. But if we walk in the light, as he is in the light, we have fellowship with one another, and the blood of Jesus, his Son, purifies us from all sin. If we claim to be without sin, we deceive ourselves and the truth is not in us.

**1 John 5:4** For everyone born of God overcomes the world. This is the victory that has overcome the world, even our faith.

**1 John 5:14** This is the assurance we have in approaching God: that if we ask anything according to his will, he hears us.

**3 John 2** Dear friend, I pray that you may enjoy good health and that all may go well with you, even as your soul is getting along well.

**1 John 3:8** He who does what is sinful is of the devil, because the devil has been sinning from the beginning. The reason the Son of God appeared was to destroy the devil's work.

**Psalm 30:5** For his anger lasts only a moment, but his favor lasts a lifetime; weeping may remain for a night, but rejoicing comes in the morning.

**Hebrews 11:6** And without faith it is impossible to please God, because anyone who comes to him must believe that he exists and that he rewards those who earnestly seek him.

**Romans 2:11** For God does not show favoritism.

**Hebrews 10:23** Let us hold unswervingly to the hope we profess, for he who promised is faithful

**Isaiah 43:1–2** But now, this is what the Lord says. He who created you, O Jacob, he who formed you, O Israel; "Fear not, for I have redeemed you; I have called you by name; you are mine. When you pass through the waters, I will be with you; and when you pass through the rivers, they will not sweep over you when you walk through the fire, you will not be burned; the flames will not set you ablaze."

**Isaiah 46:4** Even to your old age and gray hairs I am he, I am he who will sustain you. I have made you and I will carry you; I will sustain you and I will rescue you.

**Psalm 119:92–93** If your law had not been my delight, I would have perished in my affliction. I will never forget your precepts, for by them you have renewed my life.

**Psalm 118:6–7** The Lord is with me, I will not be afraid. What can man do to me? The Lord is with me; he is my helper. I will look in triumph on my enemies.

**Psalm 37:3–8** Trust in the Lord and do good; dwell in the land and enjoy safe pasture. Delight yourself in the Lord and he will give you the desires of your heart. Commit your way to the Lord; trust in him and he will do this; he will make your righteousness shine like the dawn, the justice of your cause like the noonday sun.

**Isaiah 55:10–11** Though the mountains be shaken and the hills be removed, yet my unfailing love for you will not be shaken nor my covenant of peace be removed says the Lord who has compassion on you. O afflicted city, lashed by storms and not comforted, I will build you with stones of turquoise, your foundations with sapphires.

**Proverbs 12:18** Reckless words pierce like a sword, but the tongue of the wise brings healing.

**Proverbs 16:24** Pleasant words are a honeycomb, sweet to the soul and healing to the bones.

**Proverbs 13:3** He who guards his lips guards his soul, but he who speaks rashly will come to ruin.

**Proverbs 18:21** The tongue has the power of life and death, and those who love it will eat its fruit.

**John 17:17** Sanctify them by truth; your word is truth.

**Psalm 141:3** Set a guard over your mouth, O Lord keep watch over the door of my lips

**James 1:4–7** Perseverance must finish its work so that you may be mature and complete, not lacking anything. If any of you lacks wisdom, he should ask God, who gives generously to all without finding fault, and it will be given to him. But when he asks, he must believe and not doubt, because he who doubts is like the wave of the sea, blown and tossed by the wind. That man should not think he will receive anything from the Lord.

**Luke 10:19** I have given you authority to trample on snakes and scorpions and to overcome all the power of the enemy; nothing will harm you.

**Ephesians 6:11–13** Put on the full armor of God so that you can take your stand against the devil's schemes. For our struggle is not against flesh and blood, but against the authorities, against the powers of this dark world and against the spiritual forces of evil in the heavenly realms. Therefore, put on the full armor of God, so that when the day of evil comes, you may be able to stand your ground, and after you have done everything, to stand.

# Cancer Is Limited

*It cannot cripple love,*
*It cannot shatter hope,*
*It cannot corrode faith,*
*It cannot eat away at peace,*
*It cannot destroy confidence,*
*It cannot shut out memories*
*It cannot silence courage,*
*It cannot invade the soul,*
*It cannot reduce eternal life,*
*It cannot quench the spirit,*
*It cannot lessen the power of the Resurrection.*

Blessed Sacrament Church
Seattle, Washington

# Detoxification Techniques: Some Friendly Advice

**1. The Famous and Therapeutic Coffee Enema**

Supply List:
- Organic ground coffee, not decaffeinated or instant
- Glass or stainless cooking pot
- Stainless steel strainer
- Enema bag or bucket (I prefer a bucket, which is easy to clean and reuse)
- Clothes hanger or wall hook
- Distilled water
- Acidophilus and or bifidophilus replacement
- Electrolyte or mineral supplements

Preparing the Coffee:

Use 3 tablespoons coffee to each quart of water. Prepare enough coffee for the day. Reduce the water during heating. Then add room-temperature water to cool down the solution for quicker use. Bring water and coffee to a boil, then reduce and simmer 20 minutes.

Strain grounds out, and prepare for one enema. Add 2 cups of coffee mixture to enema delivery bucket.

Preparation and Application:
- A bathroom is a good location for the enema process.
- Pour coffee into the enema bag or bucket and close clamp.
- Attach a clothes hanger or hook to the wall or towel rack to suspend the bag or bucket at a height of about 36–40 inches.
- Release clamp and allow coffee to begin to remove air along tubing; clamp when coffee begins to come out.
- Place a large plastic bag on the floor covered by an old blanket (for comfort) then another plastic barrier, then a towel.
- Apply lubricant to tip and lie on your back and allow the coffee to flow in. Massage abdomen from the right side to the left. After 5 minutes lie on the right side; retain coffee for 15–20 minutes total.
- Release coffee into the toilet and clean up. Use rubbing alcohol or bleach to sanitize everything. Clean thoroughly with hot soapy water after sanitizing.

## 2. Sauna Regimen

The sauna therapy causes the body to release toxins—which are stored in the fat reserves—and converts these fat soluble chemicals into water-soluble chemicals, so they can be eliminated by the body through skin, liver, kidneys, and intestines.

    The length of the sauna will vary from person to person and should be monitored carefully. Initially, in the detox center I did three hours of sauna per day but had direct supervision with constant monitoring. At home I now do three to five hours per week. I set the temperature between 135–140 degrees. After one of hour of sauna I get out, shower off and rest for at least 15 minutes before I start the next round. To avoid dehydration, it is imperative to drink lots of fluids and to replace electrolytes during the sauna. I found it very important to eat plenty of protein during this thermal temperature challenge to my body. Initially I lost weight and found I needed to supplement with minerals, vitamins and a good whey protein powder. At the conclusion of my sauna time, I would then take a coffee enema. At night before retiring, I would fix a psyllium and bentonite drink (Sonne's products #7 & 9), which would help to bind and carry away any toxins that were dumping into the intestinal track.

**3. Hydrotherapy at Home** (from *Healing Naturally*)

External hydrotherapy has been used throughout history to treat disease and injury. The contrast therapies, which are those that alternate between hot and cold, are effective in stimulating the immune system. They also stimulate adrenal glands, reduce congestion, alleviate inflammation and generally activate organ function. By stimulating the entire circulation in the digestive areas and the pelvis, it improves the detoxifying capability of the liver.

Supplies:
- 5 hand towels, folded in half
- 1 Bath mat, folded in half
- 1 full-size sheet
- 2 full-size wool blankets
- pan for hot water
- pan for ice and cold water

Step 1
- Take temperature

Step 2
- Place 2 very hot towels, one on top of another, onto the chest and upper abdomen area

- Cover those towels with a dry towel
- Wrap yourself from feet to neck in sheet and blanket
- Time this process for 4 minutes

NOTE: If temperature was less than 97:
- Remove dry towel
- Place another hot towel on top of other towels and flip
- Remove the top towel
- Place dry towel back on top
- Wrap from feet to neck in sheet and blanket
- Leave on for an additional 2 minutes

Step 3
- Unwrap sheets and blankets
- Remove the dry towel
- Place a very hot towel on top of first 2 towels
- Flip all towels
- Immediately follow with an ice cold towel
- Flip
- Remove all but the cold towel
- Cover with a dry towel
- Wrap body in sheet and wool blanket from feet to neck
- Add another wool blanket (folded in half) over chest and abdominal area
- Time for 10 minutes

- After 10 minutes feel between the 2 blankets; if still cold, leave on for another 2 minutes (can do for a total of 14 minutes on this step).

Back

- Repeat steps 2 and 3 from above, omitting the NOTE instruction

After I completed my six weeks of intensive therapy (thermal therapy, sauna and colonics daily), I continued on with the therapy at home three times per week. As I continued to improve, I reduced the time to one to two times per week.

---

[1] Patrick Quillin, Ph.D., R.D., Healing Nutrients (Chicago: Contemporary Books, 1987), page 127.

[2] Max Gerson, M.D., A Cancer Therapy: Results of Fifty Cases (Bonita, CA: The Gerson Institute, 1990), pg. 16.

[3] Linda Rector-Page, N.D., Ph.D., Healthy Healing (Sacramento, CA: Spilmen Printing Co., 1990), page 32.

[4] Anne Frahm, Cancer Battle Plan (Colorado Springs, CO: Ninon Press, 1992), pg. 102.

[5] Craig Hill, The Ancient Paths (Family Foundations Publishing, 1992), pg.59-60.

# Recommended Reading and References

Anderson, Neil. *The Bondage Breaker* (Harvest House Publishers, Eugene, Oregon, 1990).

Bach, James F & Phyllis. *Prescription for Nutritional Healing* (Avery Publishing Group Inc., 1990).

Bieler, Henry. *Food Is Your Best Medicine* (Ballantine Books, New York, 1987).

Bubeck, Mark. *Overcoming the Adversary* (Moody Press, Chicago, 1989).

Bubeck, Mark. *The Adversary* (Moody Press, Chicago, 1992).

Dobson, James. *When God Doesn't Make Sense* (Tyndale House Publishers, Inc., Wheaton, Illinois, 1993).

Fink, John. *Third Opinion* (Avery Publishing Group Inc., Garden City Park, NY, 1988).

Frahm, Anne and David. *The Cancer Battle Plan* (Pinon Press, Colorado Springs, CO, 1993).

Gerson, Max. *A Cancer Therapy* (The Gerson Institute, Bonita, CA, 1990).

Gittleman, Ann Louise. *Guess What Came To Dinner* (Avery Publishing Group Inc., Garden City Park, New York).

Glassman, Judith. *The Cancer Survivors* (The Dial Press, New York, 1983).

Goldberg, Burton. *Alternative Medicine* (Future Medicine Publishing, Inc., Tiburon, California, 1999).

Gorman, Carolyn. *Less-Toxic Alternatives* (Optimum Publishing, Texarkana, Texas, 1997).

Hill, Craig. *The Ancient Paths* (Family Foundations Publishing, Littleton, CO, 1992).

Howell, Edward. *Enzyme Nutrition* (Avery Publishing Group Inc., Wayne, New Jersey, 1985).

Hunsberger, Eydie Mae. *How I Conquered Cancer Naturally* (Avery Publishing Group Inc., Garden City Park, New York, 1992).

Jensen, Bernard. *Tissue Cleansing Through Bowel Management* (Bernard Jensen, D.C., Escondido, CA, 1981).

Josephson, Elmer A. *God's Key to Health and Happiness* (Fleming H. Revell, A Division of Baker Book House, Grand Rapids, Michigan 1976).

LeShan, Lawrence. *You Can fight For Your Life* (M. Evans and Company, Inc., New York, 1977).

Lopez, Williams Miehlke. *Enzymes the Fountain of Life* (Neville Press, Inc., Charleston, SC, 1994).

Matsen, John. *Eating Alive, Prevention through Good Digestion* (Crompton Books Ltd., North Vancouver, BC, 1991).

McMillen, S.I.M. *None of These Diseases* (Fleming H. Revell Co., Old Tappan, New Jersey, 1984).

Pert, Candace B. *Molecules of Emotion* (Simon and Schuster, Rockefeller Center, New York, NY, 1997).

Quillin, Patrick. *Healing Nutrients* (Random House, New York, 1989.)

Rector-Page, Linda. *Healthy Healing* (Healthy Healing Publications, 1992).

Salaman, Maureen. *The Cancer Answer* (Statford Publishing, 1259 El Camino Real, Suite 1500, Menlo Park, CA).

Sandford, John and Paula. *The Transformation of the Inner Man* (Bridge Publishing, Inc., So. Plainfield, NJ, 1982).

Sandford, John and Mark. *Deliverance and Inner Healing* (Chosen Books, Baker Book House Co., Grand Rapids, Michigan, 1992).

Seamands, David. *Putting Away Childish Things* (Victor Books, a division of SP publications, Inc., Wheaton, Illinois, 1984).

Siegel, Bernie S. *Love, Medicine and Miracles* (Harper and Row, Publishers, New York, 1990).

Wigmore, Ann. *The Sprouting Book* (Avery Publishing Group Inc., Wayne, New Jersey, 1986).

Wigmore, Ann. *The Wheatgrass Book* (Avery Publishing Group Inc., Wayne, New Jersey, 1986).

Williams, Linsey. *You Can Live Life and Health* Publication, Portland, Oregon, 1989).

Williams, Roger. *Nutrition Against Disease* (Pitman Publishing Corporation, New York, N.Y., 1980).

Yancey, Philip. *Where Is God When It Hurts?* (Zondervan Publishing House, Grand Rapids, Michigan, 1990).

To order additional copies of

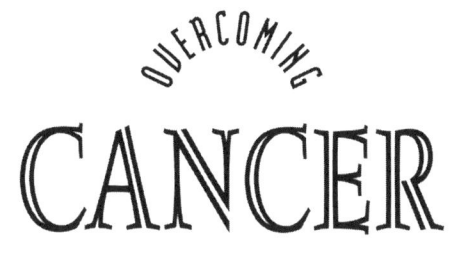

# OVERCOMING CANCER
## Exposing Toxic Enemies of the Spirit, Soul, and Body

Have your credit card ready and call

toll free (877) 421-READ (7323)

or send $10.99* each plus S4.95 S&H**

to

WinePress Publishing
PO Box 428
Enumclaw, WA 98022

www.winepresspub.com

*WA residents, add 8.4% sales tax

** Add $1.00 S&H for each additional book ordered.